Evidence-Based Practices
in Mental Health Care

Evidence-Based Practices in Mental Health Care

Edited by

Robert E. Drake, M.D., Ph.D.
Howard H. Goldman, M.D., Ph.D.

A Compendium of Articles From *Psychiatric Services*

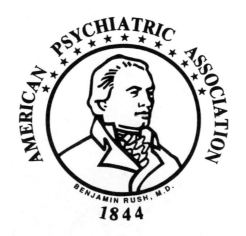

Note: The authors have worked to ensure that all information in this book is accurate at the time of publication and consistent with general psychiatric and medical standards, and that information concerning drug dosages, schedules, and routes of administration is accurate at the time of publication and consistent with standards set by the U.S. Food and Drug Administration and the general medical community. As medical research and practice continue to advance, however, therapeutic standards may change. Moreover, specific situations may require a specific therapeutic response not included in this book. For these reasons and because human and mechanical errors sometimes occur, we recommend that readers follow the advice of physicians directly involved in their care or the care of a member of their family.

The findings, opinions, and conclusions of this report do not necessarily represent the views of the officers, trustees, or all members of the American Psychiatric Association. The views expressed are those of the authors of the individual chapters.

Manufactured in the United States of America on acid-free paper
06 05 04 03 4 3
First Edition

Originally published in *Psychiatric Services,* Volumes 52 and 53

American Psychiatric Association
1000 Wilson Boulevard
Arlington, VA 22209-3901
www.psych.org

Library of Congress Cataloging-in-Publication Data
Evidence-based practices in mental health care.
     p. cm.
  Include bibliographical references.
  ISBN 0-89042-294-X (alk. paper)
  1. Mental health services. 2. Evidence-based medicine. I. American Psychiatric
Association.

  RA790.5.E843 2003
  362.2'1—dc21

                                                                    2002043870

British Library Cataloguing in Publication Data
A CIP record is available from the British Library.

Contents

Introduction vii
Robert E. Drake, M.D., Ph.D., and Howard H. Goldman, M.D., Ph.D.

Implementing Evidence-Based Practices in Routine Mental Health Service Settings 1
*Robert E. Drake, M.D., Ph.D., Howard H. Goldman, M.D., Ph.D., H. Stephen Leff, Ph.D., Anthony
F. Lehman, M.D., M.P.H., Lisa Dixon, M.D., M.P.H., Kim T. Mueser, Ph.D., and William C. Torrey, M.D.*

Implementing Evidence-Based Practices for Persons With Severe Mental Illnesses 5
*William C. Torrey, M.D., Robert E. Drake, M.D., Ph.D., Lisa Dixon, M.D., M.P.H., Barbara J. Burns,
Ph.D., Laurie Flynn, A. John Rush, M.D., Robin E. Clark, Ph.D., and Dale Klatzker, Ph.D.*

Strategies for Disseminating Evidence-Based Practices to Staff Who
Treat People With Serious Mental Illness 11
*Patrick W. Corrigan, Psy.D., Leigh Steiner, Ph.D., Stanley G.
McCracken, Ph.D., Barbara Blaser, R.N., and Michael Barr, Ph.D.*

Integrating Evidence-Based Practices and the Recovery Model 21
Frederick J. Frese III, Ph.D., Jonathan Stanley, J.D., Ken Kress, J.D., Ph.D., and Suzanne Vogel-Scibilia, M.D.

Implementing Supported Employment as an Evidence-Based Practice 29
*Gary R. Bond, Ph.D., Deborah R. Becker, M.Ed., Robert E. Drake, M.D., Ph.D., Charles A. Rapp, Ph.D.,
Neil Meisler, M.S.W., Anthony F. Lehman, M.D., M.S.P.H., Morris D. Bell, Ph.D., and Crystal R. Blyler, Ph.D.*

Implementing Dual Diagnosis Services for Clients With Severe Mental Illness 39
*Robert E. Drake, M.D., Ph.D., Susan M. Essock, Ph.D., Andrew Shaner, M.D.,
Kate B. Carey, Ph.D., Kenneth Minkoff, M.D., Lenore Kola, Ph.D., David Lynde,
M.S.W., Fred C. Osher, M.D., Robin E. Clark, Ph.D., and Lawrence Rickards, Ph.D.*

Moving Assertive Community Treatment Into Standard Practice 47
*Susan D. Phillips, M.S.W., Barbara J. Burns, Ph.D., Elizabeth R. Edgar, M.S.S.W., Kim T. Mueser, Ph.D., Karen W.
Linkins, Ph.D., Robert A. Rosenheck, M.D., Robert E. Drake, M.D., Ph.D., and Elizabeth C. McDonel Herr, Ph.D.*

Evidence-Based Practices for Services to Families of People With Psychiatric Disabilities 57
*Lisa Dixon, M.D., M.P.H., William R. McFarlane, M.D., Harriet Lefley, Ph.D.,
Alicia Lucksted, Ph.D., Michael Cohen, M.A., Ian Falloon, M.D., Kim Mueser, Ph.D.,
David Miklowitz, Ph.D., Phyllis Solomon, Ph.D., and Diane Sondheimer, M.S., M.P.H.*

Evidence-Based Pharmacologic Treatment for People With
Severe Mental Illness: A Focus on Guidelines and Algorithms 65
*Thomas A. Mellman, M.D., Alexander L. Miller, M.D., Ellen M. Weissman, M.D.,
M. Lynn Crismon, Pharm.D., Susan M. Essock, Ph.D., and Stephen R. Marder, M.D.*

Developing Effective Treatments for Posttraumatic
Disorders Among People With Severe Mental Illness 73
Stanley D. Rosenberg, Ph.D., Kim T. Mueser, Ph.D., Matthew J. Friedman, M.D., Ph.D., Paul G. Gorman, Ed.D.,
Robert E. Drake, M.D., Ph.D., Robert M. Vidaver, M.D., William C. Torrey, M.D., and Mary K. Jankowski, Ph.D.

Evidence-Based Practice in Child and Adolescent Mental Health Services 83
Kimberly Hoagwood, Ph.D., Barbara J. Burns, Ph.D., Laurel Kiser,
Ph.D., Heather Ringeisen, Ph.D., and Sonja K. Schoenwald, Ph.D.

Evidence-Based Practices in Geriatric Mental Health Care 95
Stephen J. Bartels, M.D., Aricca R. Dums, B.A., Thomas E. Oxman, M.D., Lon S. Schneider,
M.D., Patricia A. Areán, Ph.D., George S. Alexopoulos, M.D., and Dilip V. Jeste, M.D.

Policy Implications for Implementing Evidence-Based Practices 109
Howard H. Goldman, M.D., Ph.D., Vijay Ganju, Ph.D., Robert E. Drake, M.D., Ph.D.,
Paul Gorman, Ed.D., Michael Hogan, Ph.D., Pamela S. Hyde, J.D., and Oscar Morgan

Introduction

Robert E. Drake, M.D., Ph.D.
Howard H. Goldman, M.D., Ph.D.

The evidence-based-practices movement has become a catalyst for reform in the public mental health system. National organizations and state mental health systems alike have embraced the concept that they have an ethical obligation to provide treatments that work.

One question that arises is, Why now? The U.S. health care system has been committed to scientifically based treatment for the past century, and the movement to adopt a set of specific techniques in general medicine, which is termed evidence-based medicine, is now more than a decade old (1). A confluence of several developments may have created the impetus for change. The evidence base regarding effective treatments for persons with severe mental illness who are living in the community in the postdeinstitutionalization era has been steadily building for nearly 50 years. The Schizophrenia Patient Outcomes Research Team project (2) was seminal in clarifying that we know a considerable amount about treatments that work and that these treatments are not widely available and used. The Surgeon General's first report on mental illness clarified these points for the public (3).

With the crisis in health care funding and the movement toward managed care, the demand for accountability has been pervasive. The courts have ruled repeatedly that mental health care providers have a legal obligation to provide the best available treatments. The National Alliance for the Mentally Ill, the National Association for State Mental Health Program Directors, the Robert Wood Johnson Foundation, the MacArthur Foundation, the West Foundation, and other national organizations and advocacy groups in one way or another have provided support and leadership in the movement toward effective treatment. The National Institute of Mental Health has shifted its research emphasis to study treatments that work in routine practice settings rather than primarily in university settings. The Center for Mental Health Services of the Substance Abuse and Mental Health Services Administration has led the effort to identify and disseminate effective treatments. Remarkably, all this has happened in the context of even more limited mental health care dollars (4).

John A. Talbott, M.D., the editor of *Psychiatric Services*, has been a leader in mental health care reform for decades. When we approached him about publishing a series on this topic for the journal, he immediately recognized the timeliness and significance of the issue. The papers in this volume were originally published in *Psychiatric Services* during 2001 and 2002. They are remarkable in representing a broad-based attempt to synthesize the available information on the effectiveness of community-based mental health practices. Several papers address general issues in the field: What do we know about reviewing the evidence transparently, about implementing practices in routine mental health settings, and about the policy implications of this movement?

Other papers address specific practices for which substantial evidence exists, including practices for particular populations.

The field of evidence-based mental health practices is in its infancy. These initial attempts to summarize the knowledge and issues are ungainly in many ways. The common criticisms of evidence-based practices—for example, that they conflict with recovery and other ideological commitments—highlight the inadequate job we have done to inform all stakeholders about the philosophy of evidence-based medicine and developments in the mental health field. The basic tenets of evidence-based medicine have not been articulated and discussed in public forums. We have not clarified several issues. For example, we need to demonstrate how scientific evidence can be used to improve the quality of services and the quality of life of service recipients as well as how a hierarchy of evidence is constructed and used in decision making. We also need to clarify how other important issues, such as individual client characteristics, client preferences for treatment and outcomes, and client autonomy, are valued in evidence-based practices (5).

Consumers and families have expressed fears that they will be displaced from their roles in delivering services and supports, that their service options and choices will be reduced, and that services will be less individualized. All these fears are in fact antithetical to the basic tenets of evidence-based practices. Practitioners have expressed concerns about the credibility of the evidence base, the difficulty of learning new techniques and taking on new responsibilities without training and time, and the lack of inclusion of their favorite interventions in the initial attempts to

Dr. Drake is professor of psychiatry at Dartmouth Medical School and director of the New Hampshire–Dartmouth Psychiatric Research Center in Lebanon, New Hampshire. Dr. Goldman is professor of psychiatry at the University of Maryland School of Medicine in Baltimore.

identify evidence-based practices. Administrators and policy makers have also expressed concerns, often related to the difficulties of financing, organizing, implementing, and sustaining new practices. Vested-interest groups feel a new pressure to show that what they do is effective.

All these concerns should be discussed publicly. Without public debate, evidence-based practices, as has been the case with some other attempts at reform, could be transmogrified into unintended representa-

tions and conclusions that might further restrict access to effective and needed care. Thus we consider these articles to be a starting point. It has been our privilege to bring these papers together. It is our hope that they will stimulate helpful discussion. ♦

References

1. Evidence-Based Medicine Working Group: Evidence-based medicine: a new approach to teaching the practice of medicine. JAMA 268:2420–2425, 1992

2. Lehman AF, Steinwachs DM, Survey Co-Investigators of the PORT Project: Translating research into practice: the Schizophrenia Patient Outcomes Research Team (PORT) treatment recommendations. Schizophrenia Bulletin 24:1–10, 1998

3. Mental Health: A Report of the Surgeon General. Washington, DC, Department of Health and Human Services, US Public Health Service, 2000

4. Appelbaum PS: Starving in the midst of plenty: the mental health care crisis in America. Psychiatric Services 53:1247–1248, 2002

5. Haynes RB, Devereaux PJ, Guyatt GH: Clinical expertise in the era of evidence-based medicine and patient choice. ACP (American College of Physicians) Journal Club, Mar–Apr 2002, p A11

Implementing Evidence-Based Practices in Routine Mental Health Service Settings

Robert E. Drake, M.D., Ph.D.
Howard H. Goldman, M.D., Ph.D.
H. Stephen Leff, Ph.D.
Anthony F. Lehman, M.D., M.P.H.
Lisa Dixon, M.D., M.P.H.
Kim T. Mueser, Ph.D.
William C. Torrey, M.D.

The authors describe the rationale for implementing evidence-based practices in routine mental health service settings. Evidence-based practices are interventions for which there is scientific evidence consistently showing that they improve client outcomes. Despite extensive evidence and agreement on effective mental health practices for persons with severe mental illness, research shows that routine mental health programs do not provide evidence-based practices to the great majority of their clients with these illnesses. The authors define the differences between evidence-based practices and related concepts, such as guidelines and algorithms. They discuss common concerns about the use of evidence-based practices, such as whether ethical values have a role in shaping such practices and how to deal with clinical situations for which no scientific evidence exists.

An important focus of *Psychiatric Services* in 2001 is on the implementation of evidence-based interventions in mental health care. In last month's issue (1), the journal initiated a series of papers on implementing evidence-based practices for the care of persons with severe mental illnesses in routine mental health service settings. Papers in this series will describe the conceptual framework of a national demonstration project, the Evidence-Based Practices Project, which is sponsored by the Robert Wood Johnson Foundation, the Center for Mental Health Services of the Substance Abuse and Mental Health Services Administration, the National Alliance for the Mentally Ill, and several mental health research centers, state mental health authorities, and local mental health programs in New Hampshire, Maryland, Ohio, North Carolina, and Texas.

The goal of the project is to develop standardized guidelines and training materials, in the form of toolkits, and to demonstrate that the toolkits can be used to facilitate the faithful implementation of evidence-based practices and to improve client outcomes in routine mental health service settings.

In this paper we present the concept of evidence-based practices. We describe the background of the movement toward such practices and define evidence-based practices and related concepts. We also discuss common concerns about the use of evidence-based practices in routine mental health service settings.

The rationale for evidence-based practices

Psychiatric Services' decision to dedicate 2001 to evidence-based practices rests on a series of research findings and philosophical commitments. First, a great deal is now known about efficacious and effective mental health interventions, which we refer to here as evidence-based practices. For example, numerous research reviews identify a core set of interventions that help persons with severe mental illness attain better outcomes in terms of symptoms, functional status, and quality of life (2–6). The core set includes medications prescribed within specific parameters, training in illness self-management, assertive community treatment, family psychoeducation, supported employment, and integrated treatment for co-occurring substance use disorders (7). In upcoming issues, experts will review research evidence on outcomes, present current knowl-

Dr. Drake and Dr. Mueser are professors of psychiatry and Dr. Torrey is associate professor of psychiatry at the New Hampshire–Dartmouth Psychiatric Research Center, 2 Whipple Place, Lebanon, New Hampshire 03766 (robert.e.drake@dartmouth.edu). Dr. Leff is assistant professor of psychiatry at Harvard Medical School and at the Cambridge Hospital in Cambridge, Massachusetts. Dr. Goldman and Dr. Lehman are professors of psychiatry and Dr. Dixon is associate professor of psychiatry at the University of Maryland School of Medicine in Baltimore. This article was originally published in the February 2001 issue of Psychiatric Services.

edge about barriers and strategies related to implementation, and discuss implications.

A second reason for the journal's focus on evidence-based practices is that despite extensive evidence and agreement on effective mental health practices for persons with severe mental illness, research also shows that routine mental health programs do not provide evidence-based practices to most clients with these illnesses (8). This finding was a major conclusion of the report of the Surgeon General (6). In the most extensive demonstration of this problem, the Schizophrenia Patient Outcomes Research Team showed that in two state mental health systems, clients with a diagnosis of schizophrenia were highly unlikely to receive effective services (9). For example, antipsychotic medications were often prescribed at dosages outside the effective range. A minority of clients—often as few as 10 percent—received evidence-based psychosocial services, such as family interventions. Findings from other sources suggest a dearth of evidence-based practices in routine mental health settings (10).

Third, research indicates that offering a service that resembles an evidence-based practice is not sufficient; adherence to specific programmatic standards, often referred to as fidelity of implementation, is necessary to produce expected outcomes (11–13). In other words, if two programs offer a practice of care that is known to be effective, the program with higher fidelity to the defined practice model tends to produce superior outcomes. This critical finding, which contradicts the conventional wisdom that model programs do not transfer and need to be modified extensively to fit local circumstances, suggests that implementation guidelines and toolkits should begin to incorporate manuals and fidelity measures (14).

Fourth, mental health services for persons with severe mental illness should reflect the goals of consumers. People with severe mental illness, like people with other long-term illnesses, want to pursue normal, functional, satisfying lives to the greatest extent possible (15,16). Mental health services therefore should not focus exclusively on traditional outcomes of treatment compliance and prevention of relapses and rehospitalizations. The new paradigm emphasizes helping people attain outcomes such as independence, employment, satisfying relationships, and good quality of life.

Fifth, given that mental health resources are limited, persons with severe mental illness have a right to have access to interventions that are known to be effective and that are delivered in a manner faithful to or consistent with current understandings of the interventions' active ingredients. In other words, to the extent that evidence-based practices exist, they should be the bedrock, the minimum of acceptable offerings, in all mental health settings that provide services for persons with severe mental illness. Additional services may enhance the service offering and may prove to be effective over time, but the basic offering of evidence-based practices should not be displaced by interventions of unknown or lesser effectiveness. Researchers, state mental health directors, consumers, and families support this commitment and have endorsed the urgent need for dissemination and implementation of evidence-based practices (17).

Finally, evidence-based practices do not provide the answers for all persons with mental illness, all outcomes, or all settings. Below we discuss several caveats as well as the judicious and informed use of evidence-based practices. Accurate information about effective practices, including a clear understanding of the limitations of current research and the need for further evidence in many areas, can improve services and outcomes. However, to produce positive changes, the research evidence on effective services and the implementation procedures must be available to all stakeholders in the service system (1).

What are evidence-based practices?
Evidence-based practices are interventions for which there is consistent scientific evidence showing that they improve client outcomes. For example, research shows that using antipsychotic medications within specific dosage ranges and providing education and skill training for family caregivers over several months prevents or delays relapses of schizophrenia (4). The requirements for scientific evidence used by different groups sometimes vary, but in general the highest standard is several randomized clinical trials comparing the practice to alternative practices or to no intervention. When the separate trials are considered together, such as through a meta-analysis, the evidence supports the superiority of the evidence-based practice over the alternatives, including no intervention.

In some situations quasi-experimental studies, with comparison groups that are not assigned by randomization, constitute the best available evidence and consistently support a specific evidence-based practice. Rather than rigid decision rules, which inevitably are more appropriate for some types of interventions than others, we encourage panels of research scientists to review the available controlled studies and to make explicit their criteria for inclusion, the studies reviewed, the review procedures, and the conclusions so that others can examine the same evidence and reasoning.

Open clinical trials, which lack independent comparison groups, provide a significantly lower level of research evidence and are generally not considered to provide sufficiently strong scientific evidence. The lowest level of evidence, which should not be considered research evidence, consists of clinical observations collected as expert opinion. Best practices based on clinical opinions or open clinical trials do not constitute evidence-based practices, because they are not research based, are fraught with potential for error, and are often contradicted by later findings of controlled research.

Some groups, such as the Agency for Healthcare Research and Quality, have identified levels of scientific evidence, which they use to score evidence-based practices. The various practice guidelines developed in the 1990s by the agency—then known as the Agency for Health Care Policy and Research (18)—exemplify this approach by using three levels of evidence: level A refers to good research-based evidence, with some expert opinion. Level B indicates fair research-based evidence, with substantial expert opinion, to support the recommendation. Level C denotes a recommendation based primarily on expert opinion, with minimal research-based evidence.

Although the term evidence-based practice is sometimes used to refer to guidelines that are not based on research, true evidence-based practices are by definition grounded in consistent research evidence that is sufficiently specific to permit the assessment of the quality of the practices rendered as well as the outcomes. For example, supported employment is sufficiently well defined and standardized so that its fidelity can be measured and it can be differentiated from other approaches to vocational rehabilitation (14).

Other guidelines, such as those developed by the American Psychiatric Association (19), are based on a mixture of randomized clinical trials and expert consensus and often lack sufficient specificity to provide tools for judging the quality of interventions. There are also consensus guidelines, such as those developed by the triuniversity consortium (20), that systematically define desired practices through an iterative consensus process among experts. The advantage of the expert consensus approach is that it permits development of guidelines about practices for which no systematic research evidence exists. The major disadvantage is that the expert opinions may reflect current biases in the field rather than demonstrated effectiveness. At the far end of the continuum are guidelines that are written primarily to serve some administrative function and that are supported neither by research evidence nor by expert consensus.

Treatment decisions are typically complex, involving multiple decision steps that depend on the patient's response to treatment at each step. This complexity has led to the development of treatment algorithms that map out a series of decision points based on responses to the previous steps. For example, an algorithm for pharmacologic treatment of a person experiencing acute symptoms of schizophrenia may begin with initiation of an antipsychotic medication within a specific dosage range. If the person fails to respond adequately to the treatment, the algorithm may specify a second option—for example, switching to another class of antipsychotic agent. Failure to respond to the second treatment would lead to a third decision point—for example, initiation of clozapine treatment. Such algorithms may be particularly useful in guiding clinicians through a complex series of treatment decisions.

As with guidelines, algorithms may have varying levels of scientific evidence to support them. A current challenge in algorithm development is that the scientific evidence supporting the successive steps quickly becomes quite thin. Hence even the most evidence-based algorithms typically begin with steps supported by multiple clinical trials and evolve into steps defined through expert consensus. An excellent example of treatment algorithms has been developed in the Texas Medication Algorithm Project (5).

Questions about the use of evidence-based practices

A number of questions arise in relation to the recent emphasis on evidence-based practices. For example, what is the role of ethical values in shaping practices? What should be done when there are different levels of evidence or changes in evidence? What are the limits of evidence? What should be done in clinical situations for which there is no scientific evidence? We briefly address each of these points below and will do so in greater detail in upcoming issues of the journal.

Values

Mental health services appropriately incorporate humanistic values, ethical principles, and legal standards. For example, addressing adult clients as adults, interacting benignly and respectfully with families, and showing sensitivity with respect to age, sex, race, and cultural background are core values of the health care system (21). Research is not required to support these standards, and nothing about evidence-based practices contravenes the importance of such standards. On the contrary, this discussion assumes that evidence-based practices must incorporate consensual values, ethical principles, and legal standards.

Nature of the evidence

As noted, research evidence is often complicated, with inconsistent results and differences in the design, quality, and number of studies of any single intervention. Moreover, the evidence evolves rapidly. Thus the need for scientific review is critical and ongoing. For policy purposes, however, the transition from existing practices to evidence-based practices is more clear-cut. Existing practices typically rely on tradition, convenience, clinicians' preferences, political correctness, marketing, and clinical wisdom—none of which is consistently related to improving outcomes. Historically, clinical practice in mental health is often completely unhelpful and sometimes tragically harmful, as in the case of psychosurgery.

The crux of the matter is that precisely because evidence-based practices are grounded in the qualifications imposed by current science, they are standardized, replicable, and effective. A switch to research-based interventions with known effectiveness can dramatically improve outcomes in large practice systems—for example, the overall rate of employment of persons with severe mental illness (22).

Limitations of the evidence

Research evidence on interventions is often quite specific with respect to population, outcome, and context. For example, research clearly demonstrates that assertive community treatment effectively reduces hospital use for clients with schizophrenia who are unstable, homeless, treatment resistant, or hospital prone, especially in settings in which the alternative services are hospital based or clinic based (23–25). But the evidence is less clear in several areas. Does assertive community treatment improve functional outcomes such as employment? Should clients who are more stable be given assertive community treatment? What about different ethnocultural groups? What about clients with other diagnoses, such as borderline personality disorder, posttraumatic stress disorder, or substance use disorders? Is assertive community treatment needed in settings in which the usual services have incorporated its basic features such as outreach?

The central strategy in defining evidence-based practices is to be straightforward about the limits of the evidence. The provision of evidence-based practices even under circumscribed conditions would be an improvement and would move stakeholders toward awareness of the potential of other evidence-based practices. For example, research indicates that assertive community treatment does not consistently improve vocational outcomes and that supported employment must be a well-integrated component of the intervention to achieve high rates of competitive employment (25). Thus providing assertive community treatment should increase pressure to implement supported employment.

Extensions of the evidence should be careful, logical, and able to be evaluated. Because supported employment improves employment outcomes for white, African-American, and Hispanic-American clients, offering it to other cultural minorities would be a logical decision, unless there are obvious cultural differences in the meaning of work. On the other hand, logic dictates that family psychoeducation may have different meanings and effects in different cultures, and some negative research findings among Hispanic-American families (26) reinforce caution about extending the research on family psychoeducation to other groups (27).

In some situations, essentially no research exists on treatment outcomes, such as treating hepatitis C infection or the sequelae of trauma among people with severe mental illness or evaluating the effects of self-help services. The emphasis on evidence-based practices should create pressure to develop and test these interventions to fill the need for informed rather than expedient public policy. The corpus of evidence-based practices is not static, and outcomes that are valued by consumers and families should influence which interventions are developed and studied.

Conclusions

For each area of evidence-based practices, implementation in routine mental health practice settings is complex and difficult (1). Issues of organizational structure and commitment, resource development, and clarity of roles and responsibilities must be addressed before training can be effective (28). Service boundaries are often involved as well. For example, supported employment involves the interface between clinical and rehabilitative services, and dual diagnosis services highlight differences between the mental health and substance abuse treatment systems. Upcoming articles in *Psychiatric Services* will address implementation barriers and strategies as well as the specific evidence, including boundaries and extensions, for each of several evidence-based practices. Emphasis on evidence-based practices also has implications for public policy, education, research, medical information systems, managed care, liability, and many other topics. ◆

References

1. Torrey WC, Drake RE, Dixon L, et al: Implementing evidence-based practices for persons with severe mental illnesses. Psychiatric Services 52:45–50, 2001

2. Fenton WE, Schooler NR: Editor's introduction: evidence-based psychosocial treatment for schizophrenia. Schizophrenia Bulletin 26:1–3, 2000

3. Kane JM: Pharmacologic treatment of schizophrenia. Biological Psychiatry 46:1396–1408, 1999

4. Lehman AF, Steinwachs DM, Survey Co-Investigators of the PORT Project: Translating research into practice: the Schizophrenia Patient Outcomes Research Team (PORT) treatment recommendations. Schizophrenia Bulletin 24:1–10, 1998

5. Miller AL, Chiles JA, Chiles JK, et al: The Texas Medication Algorithm Project (TMAP) schizophrenia algorithms. Journal of Clinical Psychiatry 60:649–657, 1999

6. Mental Health: A Report of the Surgeon General. Washington, DC, Department of Health and Human Services, US Public Health Service, 2000

7. Drake RE, Mueser KT, Torrey WC, et al: Evidence-based treatment of schizophrenia. Current Psychiatry Reports 2:393–397, 2000

8. Leff HS, Mulkern V, Lieberman M, et al: The effects of capitation on service access, adequacy, and appropriateness. Administration and Policy in Mental Health 21:141–160, 1994

9. Lehman AF, Steinwachs DM, Survey Co-Investigators of the PORT Project: Patterns of usual care for schizophrenia: initial results from the schizophrenia Patient Outcomes Research Team (PORT) client survey. Schizophrenia Bulletin 24:11–20, 1998

10. Dixon L, Lyles A, Scott J, et al: Services to families of adults with schizophrenia: from treatment recommendations to dissemination. Psychiatric Services 50:233–238, 1999

11. Jerrel JM, Ridgely MS: Impact of robustness of program implementation on outcomes of clients in dual diagnosis programs. Psychiatric Services 50:109–112, 1999

12. McDonnell J, Nofs D, Hardman M, et al: An analysis of the procedural components of supported employment programs associated with employment outcomes. Journal of Applied Behavior Analysis 22:417–428, 1989

13. McHugo GJ, Drake RE, Teague GB, et al: Fidelity to assertive community treatment and client outcomes in the New Hampshire Dual Disorders Study. Psychiatric Services 50:818–824, 1999

14. Bond G, Williams J, Evans L, et al: Psychiatric Rehabilitation Fidelity Toolkit. Cambridge, Mass, Evaluation Center@HSRI, 2000

15. Mead S, Copeland ME: What recovery means to us: consumers' perspectives. Community Mental Health Journal 36:315–328, 2000

16. Torrey WC, Wyzik P: The recovery vision as a service improvement guide for community mental health center providers. Community Mental Health Journal 36:209–216, 2000

17. National Institute of Mental Health: Bridging Science and Service. A Report by the National Advisory Mental Health Council's Clinical Treatment and Services Research Workshop. Rockville, MD, National Institute of Mental Health, 1999

18. Depression in Primary Care. AHCPR pub 93-0550. Rockville, Md, Agency for Health Care Policy and Research, 1993

19. American Psychiatric Association: Practice Guidelines for the Treatment of Patients With Schizophrenia. Washington DC, American Psychiatric Press, 1997

20. Frances AJ, Docherty J, Kahn DA: The expert consensus guideline series: Treatment of schizophrenia. Journal of Clinical Psychiatry 57(suppl 12B):1–58, 1996

21. Culver CM, Gert B: Philosophy in Medicine. New York, Oxford Press, 1982

22. Drake RE, Fox T, Leather PK, et al: Regional variation in competitive employment for persons with severe mental illness. Administration and Policy in Mental Health 25:493–504, 1998

23. Burns BJ, Santos AB: Assertive community treatment: an update of randomized trials. Psychiatric Services 46:669–675, 1995

24. Latimer E: Economic impacts of assertive community treatment: a review of the literature. Canadian Journal of Psychiatry 44:443–454, 1999

25. Mueser KT, Bond GR, Drake RE, et al: Models of community care for severe mental illness: a review of research on case management. Schizophrenia Bulletin 24:37–74, 1998

26. Telles C, Kamo M, Mintz J, et al: Immigrant families coping with schizophrenia: behavioral family intervention v case management with a low-income Spanish speaking population. British Journal of Psychiatry 167:473–479, 1995

27. Dixon L, Adams C, Lucksted A: Update on family psychoeducation for schizophrenia. Schizophrenia Bulletin 26:5–20, 2000

28. Rapp C, Poertner J: Social Administration: A Client-Centered Approach. White Plains, NY, Longman, 1992

Implementing Evidence-Based Practices for Persons With Severe Mental Illnesses

William C. Torrey, M.D.
Robert E. Drake, M.D., Ph.D.
Lisa Dixon, M.D., M.P.H.
Barbara J. Burns, Ph.D.
Laurie Flynn
A. John Rush, M.D.
Robin E. Clark, Ph.D.
Dale Klatzker, Ph.D.

Extensive empirical research, summarized in several reviews and codified in practice guidelines, recommendations, and algorithms, demonstrates that several pharmacological and psychosocial interventions are effective in improving the lives of persons with severe mental illnesses. Yet the practices validated by research are not widely offered in routine mental health practice settings. As part of an effort to promote the implementation of evidence-based practice, the authors summarize perspectives on how best to change and sustain effective practice from the research literature and from the experiences of administrators, clinicians, family advocates, and services researchers. They describe an implementation plan for evidence-based practices based on the use of toolkits to promote the consistent delivery of such practices. The toolkits will include integrated written material, Web-based resources, training experiences, and consultation opportunities. Special materials will address the concerns of mental health authorities (funders), administrators of provider organizations, clinicians, and consumers and their families.

Practices that have been demonstrated to be effective by clinical services research could improve the lives of many people if they were widely adopted in routine health care settings. The desire to promote evidence-based practice has led to a proliferation of practice guidelines throughout medicine (1,2). As Rogers noted (3), government and professional organizations formulate guidelines "to help translate the scientific literature into concise statements intended to change practice." However, studies of the impact of practice guidelines suggest that publication and distribution of guidelines is not enough to change the practice of clinicians (2,4–6).

In the mental health field, several groups have published recommendations, guidelines, consensus statements, and treatment algorithms that are relevant to the care of adults with severe mental illnesses (7–15). Although healthy debates continue about the types and levels of research evidence, the efforts of these groups highlight the fact that much is known about how to help persons living with severe mental illnesses. For example, research strongly supports the use of specific medications prescribed in specific ways as well as the use of psychosocial interventions such as supported employment, various approaches to illness self-management, family psychoeducation, case management based on the principles of assertive community treatment, and substance abuse treatment that is integrated with mental health treatment (16).

More significant than disagreements about levels of evidence is the fact that the practices supported by research are not widely offered in routine practice settings. In the most extensive demonstration of this problem, the Schizophrenia Patient Outcome Research Team (PORT) showed that patients with a diagnosis of schizophrenia in two state mental

Dr. Torrey is associate professor of psychiatry, Dr. Drake is professor of psychiatry, and Dr. Clark is associate professor of community and family medicine and psychiatry at Dartmouth Medical School in Hanover, New Hampshire. Dr. Dixon is associate professor of psychiatry at the University of Maryland in Baltimore. Dr. Burns is professor of medical psychology at Duke University Medical Center in Durham, North Carolina. Ms. Flynn is former executive director, National Alliance for the Mentally Ill in Arlington, Virginia. Dr. Rush is professor of psychiatry at the University of Texas Southwestern Medical Center at Dallas. Dr. Klatzker is chief executive officer of the Riverbend Community Mental Health Center in Concord, New Hampshire. Address correspondence to Dr. Torrey at the New Hampshire–Dartmouth Psychiatric Research Center, 2 Whipple Place, Lebanon, New Hampshire 03301 (e-mail, william.c.torrey@dartmouth.edu). This article was originally published in the January 2001 issue of Psychiatric Services.

health systems were highly unlikely to receive effective services (17). Even simple medication practices meet standards of effectiveness about half or less than half of the time. A minority of patients—often as few as 10 percent—receive psychosocial interventions supported by effectiveness research.

Evidence from other sources supports the PORT findings. For example, Anderson and Adams (18) noted that family psychoeducation is rarely available in routine practice settings, and Tashjian and associates (19) reported that fewer than 5 percent of persons with severe mental illnesses receive supported employment services.

Thus a critical challenge for the mental health field is to facilitate the widespread adoption of research-based practices in routine mental health care settings so that persons with severe mental illnesses can benefit from services that have been shown to work (20). In this paper we review the essential ingredients of an implementation plan for evidence-based practice.

The knowledge base

This paper is part of a series of reports that stem from the Implementing Evidence-Based Practices for Severe Mental Illness Project, which is sponsored by the Robert Wood Johnson Foundation, the Center for Mental Health Services of the Substance Abuse and Mental Health Services Administration, the National Alliance for the Mentally Ill (NAMI), and state and local mental health organizations in New Hampshire, Maryland, and Ohio. The project aims to develop implementation toolkits for effective practices. Subsequent papers will describe the project in more detail and address the issue of what constitutes evidence.

To inform the design of the implementation toolkits, we assessed five complementary sources of knowledge: the literature on efforts to change practice in health care; the discussions the authors had with executive administrators from provider organizations in New Hampshire, Maryland, and Ohio during several days of meetings on implementing evidence-based practice; the findings

of focus groups with frontline clinicians who serve people with severe mental illnesses in New Hampshire and Baltimore; the advocacy experiences of NAMI; and the observations of services researchers who have implemented a range of mental health services in demonstration programs.

Research literature

Implementing a practice involves promoting change in the behavior of mental health care providers. Theorists suggest that behavior changes when intention to change is combined with the necessary skill and the absence of environmental constraint (21). Green's model (22,23) for promoting change prescribes three elements: predisposing or disseminating strategies, such as educational events or written material; enabling methods, such as practice guidelines and decision support; and reinforcing strategies, such as practice feedback mechanisms.

Research shows that education alone does not strongly influence the practice behaviors of health care providers (24–26). Additional efforts, such as increasing consumer demand for services, changing financial incentives and penalties, using administrative rules and regulations, and providing clinicians with ongoing supervision and feedback on practices, are also necessary (24,27,28). The more elements of the system of care that can be marshaled to support change and reduce resistance, the more likely practice improvements will occur. In other words, intensity of effort appears directly related to success in studies of practice change (29,30).

Furthermore, complicated changes, such as modifying the practice of a whole clinical team, require a greater intensity of effort than is needed to affect a relatively simple change, such as shifting a single prescription pattern (3,29). Guidelines are not self-implementing and must be contextualized to the actual processes of care. Sustained change requires a restructuring of the flow of the daily work so that routine procedures make it natural for the clinician to give care in the new way (31).

Katon and colleagues (32), for example, were able to improve primary care treatment of depression to con-

form to treatment guidelines developed by the Agency for Health Care Policy and Research by using an intensive, multifaceted program that included extensive physician education and restructuring of services. They found, however, that the improved care did not generalize to other depressed clinic patients seen outside the restructured intervention program, even when the patients were seen by the same physicians, and did not endure after the processes of care reverted to their previous form when the year-long intervention was complete (25).

Research also indicates that when mental health programs attempt to implement evidence-based practices, the quality of the implementation strongly influences outcomes (33–36). In other words, if two programs offer a practice of care that is known to be effective, the program that has the higher fidelity to the defined practice tends to produce superior clinical results. This finding suggests that efforts to promote evidence-based practice must include fidelity measures and self-correcting feedback mechanisms.

Implementation efforts are most effective when they address the specific needs, values, and concerns of the persons whose behavior the implementation aims to change (37,38). Specifically, administrative elements of an implementation plan must be tailored to mental health administrators, clinical training elements to clinicians, and consumer and family education to those groups.

Administrators' perspective

Mental health administrators influence the implementation of evidence-based practice by setting priorities for care and organizing the operational details of practice. During meetings with the researchers in New Hampshire and Baltimore, administrators from organizations that provide services to adults with severe mental illnesses strongly urged the development of organized resources to help programs offer evidence-based practices. Having access to clearly defined practices that are known to work and that are packaged for implementation would help administrators in their efforts to meet their responsibility to the communities they serve. High turnover of clinical staff can easily overwhelm the training resources of any one agency and underscores the need for focused, effective training materials that can be used repeatedly.

Administrators indicate that financial incentives and administrative rules and regulations must be aligned to support the implementation of evidence-based practices. The overall financing structure must be relatively stable and support the effort. To sustain evidence-based practice over time, ongoing funding must be competitive with the potential income from alternative clinical staff activities. Additional financial concerns of administrators are the cost of initial training and the cost of collecting clinical outcome data and measuring fidelity over time. Training must be efficient because the cost of training includes both the direct costs and, in fee-for-service settings, the opportunity costs of the training time. The processes for tracking clinical outcomes and practice fidelity need to be streamlined because data collection takes time and energy away from direct clinical service.

Clinicians' perspective

To understand the needs of clinicians who directly provide services to adults with severe mental illnesses, we conducted a series of seven focus groups with case managers, psychiatrists, vocational specialists, and community support program therapists from numerous practice sites in New Hampshire and Baltimore. The purpose was to ascertain what factors motivate them to change, how they learn a new practice, and what they perceive as barriers to change.

Clinicians indicated that, first, they must be convinced that the practice is worth learning; second, they need to learn a practice through observation, training, and reading; and, third, they benefit from efforts to reinforce the practice over time, such as regular supervision and feedback on activities.

Clinicians are generally not eager to change and must be convinced to adopt a new practice. In addition to

research support, they are influenced by compelling vignettes, impressions of the practice seen in action, and a practice ideology, or theory, that resonates with their values and experiences as providers. Practices that can be learned and put into action quickly are more appealing than those that require intensive learning or dramatic system change.

Clinicians are particularly motivated to learn a new practice if they believe it will help them in a clinical area where they currently feel ineffective or if they feel there will be broad consumer demand for the practice. An opportunity to discuss rationale, theory, and concerns is helpful to clinicians as they evaluate a proposed practice.

Once convinced to adopt a practice, clinicians need practical instruction. At this stage, most clinicians indicate that seeing the practice in action has more of an impact than reading about it. They endorse traveling to a training site where the practice can be observed, being visited by a skilled trainer who can demonstrate the practice, or watching instructional videotapes. Written materials complement and expand understanding gained from observing the practice. Clinicians prefer practical workbooks with clear and simple aims, principles, and examples, rather than books. The workbook should provide a clear structure of practice with examples and challenging questions. Ideally the workbook should lay out the practice in brief, easy-to-read modules allowing a clinician to read a section and immediately try the intervention.

Clinicians cite the importance of supports to consolidate and reinforce new practices. Practice-specific supervision of their clinical work is essential. Supervision helps clinicians translate the theory into daily action. Supervision can be done by an expert at a distance over the phone or, preferably, by a skilled local program leader who can motivate others to learn. Strategically placed posters listing key practice principles or relevant practice slogans support the supervision and reinforce learning through repetition. Follow-up trainings and feedback on practice are also helpful. Clinicians suggest that internet resources, advanced semi-

nars, and additional readings may all be helpful for people who have the basics and want to extend their understanding and skill.

Advocates' perspective

Advocacy can help systems move to research-based practice. For example, the National Alliance for the Mentally Ill (NAMI) has had success promoting the Program for Assertive Community Treatment (PACT). By focusing on the replication of PACT as a national priority, packaging the practice for implementation, engaging the media, coordinating NAMI state organization efforts, and communicating progress, NAMI has created a grassroots demand for PACT. Active NAMI PACT steering committees are working with providers to establish PACT in 19 states.

From the PACT dissemination effort, NAMI has learned the importance of designing communication to match the needs of the participants and reinforcing learning through repetition. NAMI created printed material to capture the attention of policy makers and administrators at the state and local levels, built information for family members into family education programs, and developed a detailed implementation manual for providers. NAMI promotes PACT at every opportunity, including media events, annual NAMI conventions, state conferences, and on the Web.

Observations of researchers

The final source of knowledge about practice implementation is the combined experience of the authors from implementing and studying medication algorithms and psychosocial interventions in routine practice settings. Our experiences make it clear that a core set of steps is required to successfully establish and maintain a desired practice. These include clearly voiced administrative support for change before training; initial clinical training using didactic methods, observation of practice, and written materials; ongoing weekly supervision by an expert, based on written principles and practices; follow-up visits by a program expert with feedback on implementation; and feedback on services and outcomes.

Model programs often dissipate after demonstration or research projects end. Practices that persist have funding and organizational structures to support the practice. These programs typically have an influential clinical or operational leader who ensures the continuity of the structures and training that maintain the practice (39–43).

Implementation toolkits

On the basis of the knowledge reviewed above, the team for the Implementing Evidence-Based Practices for Severe Mental Illness Project proposes a model for effecting change. The team will develop integrated written material, Web-based resources, training experiences, and consultation opportunities, packaged as implementation toolkits. The toolkits will be designed to promote the consistent delivery of effective services and will be developed for practices for which the evidence base is extensive and the consensus supporting the practice relatively high. The impact of the toolkits on practice will be carefully studied to learn more about how to translate research-based knowledge into practice in the care of adults with severe mental illnesses.

Clearly, practice implementation can easily fail. To succeed, the system of care must have adequate resources and be reasonably organized, and the efforts of multiple stakeholders must be aligned to support the practices. Stakeholders who play essential roles include mental health authorities (funders), who create administrative rules and financial incentives; administrators of mental health organizations, who set priorities and organize care; mental health clinicians, who provide direct care; and service consumers and their families, who create demand for and receive mental health care. The toolkits will address all of these stakeholders.

The first challenge is to predispose stakeholders to work on restructuring services. For each practice, materials will include a brief video that describes the evidence-based practice, reviews the scientific support, and provides testimony from clients and clinicians who have participated in the intervention. The video will link

the research evidence for the practice with the personal experiences of people who have benefited from receiving the intervention, thereby making the practice come to life for administrators, clinicians, and consumers and their families.

Written material for each practice will also include a list of commonly asked questions and answers, a paper summarizing the scope and limits of the evidence supporting the practice, and a general paper articulating the rationale for adopting practices that are strongly supported by research. In addition to the materials, introductory training and consensus-building group facilitation will be offered to actively engage stakeholders in the change process.

Second, once the stakeholders are predisposed to change, the toolkits will enable them to make the desired changes. For administrators of mental health authorities, implementation toolkits will include a brief document specifying the funding structures and administrative rules that create effective incentives, administrative consultation, and links to other administrators who have found mechanisms to promote specific evidence-based practices. To support change efforts by administrators of provider organizations, implementation toolkits will include general recommendations for promoting change in health care settings; a brief document that lays out recommended practice processes, such as staffing, training, meeting structure, supervision, and fidelity monitoring; and administrative consultation to help organizations overcome obstacles to establishing the practice.

Implementation toolkits for clinicians will recommend initial training, including job shadowing at a site where the practice is well established. The primary ongoing training tool will be a practical workbook that articulates the aims of the practice and the practice principles and provides clear examples. Additional supports for clinicians will include extended practice-specific supervision by trainers to help clinical supervisors learn to apply practice principles to their specific clinical dilemmas, posters articulating the practice principles, and

a Web site for the practice to link providers with other relevant research, training opportunities, and materials. For consumers and their families, a booklet will be developed that describes the practice, indicates reasonable expectations about services and outcomes, and refers people to organizations that advocate for practices, such as NAMI.

Third, once an evidence-based practice has been established, organized practice feedback will help stakeholders maintain and extend the gains. To provide system feedback, implementation toolkits will include fidelity scales for program self-assessment, simple outcome measures to track the effects of the practice, follow-up trainings either at the practice site or a training site, and a recommended process for review and revision of the implemented practice to further adapt it to site-specific circumstances and to continue to engage stakeholders in implementation.

Conclusions

Extensive empirical research demonstrates that several pharmacological and psychosocial interventions are effective in improving the lives of persons with severe mental illnesses. Despite this knowledge, there has been widespread failure to implement evidence-based practices in routine mental health settings. In this report, we have recommended ingredients of an implementation plan for evidence-based practices based on the perspectives of the research literature, administrators of provider organizations, clinicians, family advocates, and services researchers. The effectiveness of the proposed plan will be studied and the findings shared with the field. ◆

Acknowledgments

This article was supported by contract 280-00-8049 from the Center for Mental Health Services, a grant from the Robert Wood Johnson Foundation, and grants MH-00839 and MH-56147 from the National Institute of Mental Health. The authors thank Paul B. Batalden, M.D., for his comments on an earlier draft of this article.

References

1. Audet AM, Greenfield S, Field M: Medical practice guidelines: current activities and

future directions. Annals of Internal Medicine 113:709–714, 1990

2. Lomas J: Words without action? The production, dissemination, and impact of consensus recommendations. Annual Review of Public Health 12:41–65, 1991

3. Rogers EM: The challenge. lessons for guidelines from the diffusion of innovations. Journal on Quality Improvement 21:324–328, 1995

4. Cabana MD, Rand CS, Powe NR, et al: Why don't physicians follow clinical practice guidelines? A framework for improvement. JAMA 282:1458–1465, 1999

5. Kosecoff J, Kanouse DE, Rogers WH, et al: Effects of the National Institutes of Health consensus development program on physician practice. JAMA 258:2708–2713, 1987

6. Lomas J, Anderson GM, Domnick-Pierre K, et al: Do practice guidelines guide practice? The effect of a consensus statement on the practice of physicians. New England Journal of Medicine 321:1306–1311, 1989

7. American Psychiatric Association: Practice guidelines for the treatment of patients with bipolar disorder. American Journal of Psychiatry 151 (Dec suppl):1–36, 1994

8. American Psychiatric Association: Practice guidelines for the treatment of patients with schizophrenia. American Journal of Psychiatry 154 (Apr suppl):1–63, 1997

9. American Psychiatric Association: Practice guideline for the treatment of patients with major depressive disorder (revision). American Journal of Psychiatry 157 (Apr suppl):1–45, 2000

10. Crismon ML, Trivedi MH, Pigott TA, et al: The Texas Medication Algorithm Project: report of the Texas consensus conference panel on medication treatment of major depressive disorder. Journal of Clinical Psychiatry 60:142–156, 1999

11. Depression Guideline Panel: Clinical Practice Guideline, 5: Depression in Primary Care, vol 2. Treatment of Major Depression. AHCPR pub no 93-0551. Rockville, Md, Agency for Health Care Policy and Research, 1993

12. Kahn DA, Carpenter D, Frances AJ, et al: The expert consensus guideline series: treatment of bipolar disorder. Journal of Clinical Psychiatry 57 (suppl 12A):1–86, 1996

13. Lehman AF, Steinwachs DM, survey coinvestigators of the PORT project: Translating research into practice: the Schizophrenia Patient Outcomes Research Team (PORT) treatment recommendations. Schizophrenia Bulletin 24:1–10, 1998

14. McEvoy JP, Scheifler PL, Frances A (eds): The expert consensus guideline series: treatment of schizophrenia 1999. Journal of Clinical Psychiatry 60(suppl 11):1–80, 1999

15. Rush AJ, Rago WV, Crismon ML, et al: Medication treatment for the severely and persistently mentally ill: the Texas Medication Algorithm Project. Journal of Clinical Psychiatry 60:284–291, 1999

16. Drake RE, Mueser KT, Torrey WC, et al: Evidence-based treatment of schizophrenia. Current Psychiatry Reports 2:393–397, 2000

17. Lehman, AF, Steinwachs DM, survey coinvestigators of the PORT project: Patterns of usual care for schizophrenia: initial results from the Schizophrenia Patient Outcomes Research Team (PORT) client survey. Schizophrenia Bulletin 24:11–20, 1998

18. Anderson J, Adams C: Family interventions in schizophrenia: an effective but underused treatment. British Medical Journal 313:505–506, 1996

19. Tashjian M, Hayward B, Stoddard S, et al: Best Practice Study of Vocational Rehabilitation Services to Severely Mentally Ill Persons. Washington, DC, Policy Study Associates, 1989

20. Mental Health: A Report of the Surgeon General. Rockville, Md, Center for Mental Health Services, 1999

21. Fishbein M: Developing effective behavioral change interventions: some lessons learned from behavioral research, in Reviewing the Behavioral Science Knowledge Base on Technology Transfer. Edited by Backer TE, David SL, Soucy G. NIDA Research Monograph 155. Rockville Md, National Institute of Mental Health, 1995

22. Green L, Kreuter M, Deeds S, et al: Health Education Planning: A Diagnostic Approach. Palo Alto, Calif, Mayfield, 1980

23. Green L, Kreuter M: Application of Precede/Proceed in Community Settings: Health Promotion Planning: An Educational and Environmental Approach. Mountain View, Calif, Mayfield, 1991

24. Davis DA, Thomson MA, Oxman AD, et al: Changing physician performance: a systematic review of the effect of continuing medical education strategies. JAMA 274:700–705, 1995

25. Lin EH, Katon WJ, Simon GE, et al: Achieving guidelines for the treatment of depression in primary care: is physician education enough? Medical Care 35:831–842, 1997

26. Oxman AD, Thomson MA, Davis DA, et al: No magic bullets: a systematic review of 102 trials of interventions to improve professional practice. Canadian Medical Association Journal 153:1423–1431, 1995

27. Greco PJ, Eisenberg JM: Changing physician practices. New England Journal of Medicine 329:1271–1274, 1993

28. Handley MR, Stuart ME, Kirz HL: An evidence-based approach to evaluating and improving clinical practice: implementing practice guidelines. HMO Practice 8:75–83, 1994

29. Davis DA, Thomson MA, Oxman AD, et al: Evidence for the effectiveness of CME: a review of 50 randomized controlled trials. JAMA 268:1111–1117, 1992

30. Schulberg HC, Katon W, Simon GE, et al: Treating major depression in primary care practice: an update of the Agency for Health Care Policy and Research practice guidelines. Archives of General Psychiatry 55:1121–1127, 1998

31. Batalden PB, Stoltz PK: A framework for the continual improvement of health care: building and applying professional and improvement knowledge to test changes in daily work. Joint Commission Journal on Quality Improvement 19:424–445, 1993

32. Katon W, Von Korff M, Lin EHB, et al: Collaborative management to achieve treatment guidelines: impact on depression in primary care. JAMA 273:1026–1031, 1995

33. Drake RE, McHugo GJ, Becker DR, et al: The New Hampshire study of supported employment for people with severe mental illness. Journal of Consulting and Clinical Psychology 64:391–399, 1996

34. Jerrel JM, Ridgely MS: Impact of robustness of program implementation on outcomes of clients in dual diagnosis programs. Psychiatric Services 50:109–112, 1999

35. McDonnell J, Nofs D, Hardman M, et al: An analysis of the procedural components of supported employment programs associated with employment outcomes. Journal of Applied Behavioral Analysis 22:417–428, 1989

36. McHugo GJ, Drake RE, Teague GB, et al: Fidelity to assertive community treatment and client outcomes in the New Hampshire dual disorders study. Psychiatric Services 50:818–824, 1999

37. Grimshaw JM, Russell IT: Effect of clinical guidelines of medical practice: a systematic review of rigorous evaluations. Lancet 342:1317–1322, 1993

38. Soumerai SB, Avorn J: Principles of educational outreach (academic detailing) to improve clinical decision making. JAMA 263:549–556, 1990

39. Becker DR, Torrey WC, Toscano R, et al: Building recovery-oriented services: lessons from implementing IPS in community mental health centers. Psychiatric Rehabilitation Journal 22:51–54, 1998

40. Burns BJ: A call for a mental health services research agenda for youth with serious emotional disturbance. Mental Health Services Research 1:5–20, 1999

41. Liberman RP, Eckman TA: Dissemination of skills training modules to psychiatric facilities: overcoming obstacles to the utilization of a rehabilitation innovation. British Journal of Psychiatry 155(suppl 5):117–122, 1989

42. Rush AJ, Crismon ML, Toprac MG, et al: Consensus guidelines in the treatment of major depressive disorder. Journal of Clinical Psychiatry 69(suppl 20):73–84, 1998

43. Rush AJ, Crismon ML, Toprac MG, et al: Implementing guidelines and systems of care: experiences with the Texas Medication Algorithm Project (TMAP). Journal of Practical Psychiatry and Behavioral Health 5:75–86, 1999

Strategies for Disseminating Evidence-Based Practices to Staff Who Treat People With Serious Mental Illness

Patrick W. Corrigan, Psy.D.
Leigh Steiner, Ph.D.
Stanley G. McCracken, Ph.D.
Barbara Blaser, R.N.
Michael Barr, Ph.D.

Evidence-based practices have not been widely implemented in real-world treatment settings for several reasons, including existing state laws, administrative policies, funding priorities, advocates' concerns, and program staffing. Dissemination strategies focus largely on program staffing and the question of why treatment teams that are responsible for assisting people with serious mental illness fail to use evidence-based practices. In a review of the research literature, two barriers to staff dissemination emerge: individual service providers lack the necessary knowledge and skills to assimilate these practices, and certain organizational dynamics undermine the treatment teams' ability to implement and maintain innovative approaches. Three sets of strategies are useful for overcoming these barriers and fostering dissemination: packaging evidence-based practices so that specific interventions are more accessible and user-friendly to service providers; educating providers about relevant knowledge and skills; and addressing the organizational dynamics of the team to facilitate the implementation of innovations. Research on dissemination is relatively new and is less well developed than the clinical and services research enterprise that has led to evidence-based practices. Implications for future studies are discussed.

According to Goethe, "Knowing is not enough; we must apply." *Psychiatric Services*, in conjunction with the Center for Mental Health Services, the National Alliance for the Mentally Ill, and the Robert Wood Johnson Foundation, has dedicated 2001 to reviewing evidence-based practices for treating people who have a serious mental illness. The series of journal articles has reviewed empirically based practice guidelines for supported employment (1), dual diagnosis services (2), case management and assertive community treatment (3), pharmacologic treatment (4), treatment for posttraumatic stress disorders (5), and family-based services (6). The vision of these articles is clear: mental health systems must adopt evidence-based practices to ensure that an effective set of treatment services is available for people with mental illness.

This paper reviews the research on dissemination strategies that facilitate the transfer of research-based practices from academic setting to public-sector psychiatry. How does a team of diverse mental health providers develop and maintain these evidence-based practices in the real world?

There are multiple reasons why evidence-based strategies have not been implemented at satisfactory levels. These reasons reflect almost every conceivable factor that influences the provision of services: federal and state laws, local ordinances, administrative policies, funding priorities, community resources, the concerns of advocates, the interests of local consumers, and program staffing. Strategies to disseminate evidence-based practices to staff focus largely on the last factor; given that certain practices have been shown to be effective in helping some populations with specific problems, why don't treatment teams who are responsible for assisting these populations use these practices? The dissemination strategies described in our paper target this concern.

A common element of the articles in the evidence-based practices series is that services for people with serious mental illness must be based on rigorous research. Unfortunately, the effort we put into developing and evaluating treatment practices is not paralleled by the research enterprise to examine dissemination strategies. The National Institute of Mental Health recognized this concern in a 1999 program announcement for dissemination research. The institute

Dr. Corrigan, Dr. McCracken, Ms. Blaser, and Dr. Barr are with the University of Chicago Center for Psychiatric Rehabilitation, 7230 Arbor Drive, Tinley Park, Illinois 60477 (e-mail, p-corrigan@uchicago.edu). Dr. Steiner is with the Illinois Office of Mental Health. This article was originally published in the December 2001 issue of Psychiatric Services.

wanted to stimulate investigations on the array of influences that beneficially or adversely affect the adoption in practice of valid mental health research findings.

To that end, we have reviewed two strands of the literature: investigations that examine barriers to using evidence-based practices in real-world settings and studies of strategies that seek to overcome these barriers and foster the dissemination of effective practices. Although this body of investigations provides some direction for dissemination of evidence-based practices to staff, several challenges remain for future research in this area. We end the paper with a brief discussion of these challenges and directions for overcoming them.

Barriers to dissemination of evidence-based practices

Proponents of innovation are often dismayed that despite the millions of dollars and the years of effort spent in the development and evaluation of treatments for people with mental illness, service providers may take a decade or more to incorporate these treatments into their day-to-day service armamentarium (7,8). Two sets of barriers specifically related to dissemination and implementation might account for this delay.

First, individual service providers lack the basic knowledge and skills required to assimilate evidence-based practices into their regular approach to treatment. Moreover, work-related variables—for example, job burnout—undermine some staff members' interest in new and innovative practices. Second, many evidence-based practices require a team of service providers. Organizational barriers, such as poor leadership, a change-averse culture, insufficient collegial support, and bureaucratic constraints, hinder the team's effort to implement and maintain such practices.

Individual clinicians' lack of necessary knowledge and skills

Service providers who are expected to assimilate evidence-based programs into their day-to-day practice need to have mastered a basic set of competencies. Staff members who lack these skills are not able to carry out

either the simple interventions that constitute the status quo or the new ways of providing service outlined by innovative practices (9,10). Job task analyses have outlined several levels of competency that are necessary to implement the evidence-based practices that have been highlighted in the *Psychiatric Services* series (11).

Three clusters of competencies emerge from these job analyses (12, 13). First, service providers need to acquire the attitudes that are the foundation of evidence-based practices (14–16). Most important among these attitudes is a change from viewing treatment as mostly custodial—that is,

Staff members may lack the basic knowledge and skills required to assimilate evidence-based practices into their regular approach to treatment.

"the goal is to provide asylums where people with serious mental illness can live out their lives protected from their community"—to perceiving services as adjuncts to helping people regain a place in the community.

Service providers also need a broad range of knowledge to be able to assimilate evidence-based practices. Two specific knowledge bases are especially important: information about the impact of serious psychiatric disabilities—for example, psychiatric symptoms, social dysfunction, course of the disorders, and impact on family—and information about pharmacological and psychosocial interventions. Finally, service providers need to master a series of skills, basic behavioral tools that are essential for ac-

tual implementation of evidence-based practices (17). These skills include interpersonal support, instrumental support, goal setting, and skills training.

The depth and breadth of knowledge and skills needed by individual service providers will vary depending on their role in the service plan. These roles are not necessarily wedded to professional disciplines but rather represent the provider's level of responsibility in specific treatment plans. In a classic paper, Bernstein (18) made a distinction about key roles in behavior therapy that applies here. She distinguished between the behavioral engineers—experts who are charged with developing an intervention plan—and behavioral technicians—service providers who will carry out the plan.

At a minimum, behavioral technicians must have mastered the skills necessary to implement assigned components of the treatment plan. Behavioral engineers need a much broader perspective; not only must they be expert in specific skills, but they also must have mastered the range of theories that guide the specific treatment plan.

A third person has a key role in the implementation and maintenance of evidence-based practices: the individual consumer (19,20). Rather than being passive vessels of treatment, consumers of mental health services are active members of the team and take part in deciding on goals and designing interventions.

There are several reasons why individual staff members may lack the appropriate attitudes, knowledge, and skills. Some never participated in formal (preservice) training to learn them. Many staff members who provide psychosocial services to persons with mental illness have little more than a high-school education. Others receive training that is not germane to the principles and practices outlined by evidence-based practices. For example, students in some psychological training programs learn projective testing and psychodynamic therapy techniques (21,22), neither of which has been shown to be useful in treating disabilities among people with serious mental illness (23).

Training in specific disciplines may also have unintended consequences in terms of some evidence based practices (24,25). For example, rules about the kind of quantitative assessment that is fundamental to many evidence-based practices may seem incongruent with some of the basic tenets learned in nursing and medical schools (26,27). Some providers believe that quantification is contrary to care giving.

Some service providers have the necessary knowledge and skills but are unable to implement evidence-based guidelines because they are burned out. Of the various models of job burnout, the paradigm of Maslach and colleagues (28) has been especially useful for understanding the experiences of health care providers. Their model includes three components: reduced personal accomplishment, or absence of feelings of competence and success because of job stress; emotional exhaustion, or feelings of being emotionally overextended and physically drained from work; and depersonalization, or an impersonal response style to health care consumers.

Research has repeatedly shown that staff members who have high levels of emotional exhaustion and depersonalization are less likely to be aware of or implement innovative approaches to human service (29,30). Moreover, they are less interested in learning new treatment approaches, which is unfortunate, because these approaches could provide the type of knowledge and skills that would help them address work stressors and counteract burnout. Some staff members adopt an attitude that if they ignore the evidence-based treatment, it will go away.

Provider teams' difficulty in developing a cohesive service plan

Staff burnout is also associated with diminished collegial support; mental health providers who report a lack of cooperation and collaboration with peers on the treatment team are likely to be emotionally exhausted at work (31,32). Clearly, this is a troublesome phenomenon, because the success of many evidence-based practices requires the coordinated efforts of the treatment team. Assertive community treatment, services for people with dual diagnoses, and supported employment all require a multidisciplinary group of services providers who can integrate their unique skills into an effective and dynamic plan for each consumer. Service providers who are unable to work together as a team will not be able to develop a plan that is sufficiently broad to meet the exigencies of most evidence-based guidelines (33,34).

Moreover, these providers are unlikely to be able to follow a plan dynamically—that is, to change key parameters as the needs, resources, and skills of the individual consumer become more apparent. Finally, a disjointed team may not develop a collaborative relationship with the consumer but will develop instead a unilateral plan, in much the same way as the team members work with each other (19).

The research has identified several reasons—in addition to individual staff burnout—why collegial support on a treatment team fails to develop. Often, team members perceive a lack of control over programmatic decisions. They believe that service innovations, and their corresponding training initiatives, reflect the interests of the administrators rather than representing what line-level service providers believe to be the key needs and concerns of their clients (33,35). Administrative priorities are often perceived as reflecting abstract political interests rather than the more pressing needs of the team and its clients. Furthermore, treatment teams often report that their efforts are bogged down by bureaucratic constraints (33,36), including the paperwork and other documentation that are needed to track the implementation and impact of services. Staff members frequently feel that these kinds of efforts take time away from the essential aspect of their job, which is interacting with consumers.

A third variable that is critical to teamwork is leadership. Does the person who is responsible for administering the team and supervising team members have the necessary skills to do so? Two leadership styles clearly undermine teamwork. Passive management-by-exception leaders respond to organizational issues only when they arise as a barrier to performance or an exception to standard practices (37,38). This approach may be troublesome, because it focuses on staff errors. Overreliance on corrective management in the absence of positive feedback may demoralize staff. Laissez-faire leaders are uninvolved or disinterested in the day-to-day activities of their staff (39). This kind of hands-off leadership typically undermines collegiality among team members, which in turn diminishes the implementation of effective treatments.

Limited time for training

The above review clearly suggests a direction for training—namely, interventions that foster individual staff training and organizational development. Unfortunately, this need presents an interesting conundrum. The group that most requires training and development is staff who work in public-sector programs that are overwhelmed by the number of clients needing service and by the lack of resources to support these services. This group will report that more than eight hours of their workday are filled with direct service activities. How, then, can they take time away from the field to engage in training services?

Administrators will echo this concern. Service providers who are tied up in training programs are not providing billable services; hence agency income, which is already meager, is further limited. Any effort to boost the skills of individual staff and the treatment team must take this dilemma into account. In particular, training technologies that can be provided at the job site and that are quickly transferable to the practice environment have priority.

Strategies to facilitate dissemination

A variety of strategies enhance the dissemination and regular implementation of evidence-based practices. Three are reviewed here: manual- and guideline-based strategies that make evidence-based practices more user-friendly to line-level staff; education-based approaches that increase staff members' knowledge and skills; and organization-based strategies that enhance the team's ability to work collaboratively.

Making manuals and guidelines user-friendly

Some evidence-based practices have components that interfere with their transfer from the academic settings in which they were developed to real-world settings. For example, the resources and policies that foster development of an innovative practice in a research environment may not parallel the demands of consumers, providers, and administrators in the public mental health system (33). Moreover, evidence-based practices that have survived clinical trials are often steeped in jargon and principles that are unintelligible to those who do not work in academic settings (36,40). The development of treatment manuals and practice guidelines is a key strategy for making evidence-based practices more accessible to line-level staff.

Treatment manuals originally were designed to ensure that clinicians participating in efficacy studies were implementing interventions according to the protocol (41,42). These manuals spell out the specific steps through which therapists must guide consumers to accomplish the goals of the service. As the manuals were being developed, dissemination investigators realized that they provide a technology for overcoming some of the translation barriers posed by evidence-based treatments. Treatment manuals and practice guidelines have been successfully developed and disseminated for social skills training programs (43,44), family treatment (16,45), supported employment (46), and assertive community treatment (47,48).

Manuals for evidence-based treatments serve several purposes (49). The microskills contained in many treatment manuals can be quickly learned by line-level generalists, so there is no need to hire specially trained and costly professionals to implement the programs. Treatment manuals often have high face validity, which improves the likelihood that provider staff will understand the treatment's rationale and implement the technology. The manuals typically

have built-in fidelity systems that practitioners can use to ensure that they are implementing the program correctly. These systems may also include outcome assessments that assist staff in determining whether consumer goals are being accomplished.

Despite these benefits, manuals have some limitations that need to be addressed in future work. Practice guidelines and treatment manuals vary in level of detail and specific guidance. Most were not developed with the high school–educated worker as the intended provider audience and therefore require additional translation and elaboration. Manuals were

---

Treatment manuals often have high face validity, which improves the likelihood that provider staff will understand the treatment's rational and implement the technology.

---

not meant to be stand-alone dissemination strategies. Rarely do innovators believe that the information in these manuals can be implemented without some basic training. Education strategies are often combined with manuals to enhance dissemination and implementation.

Educating staff on skills and principles

Education programs target two different groups of people: those in preservice training—for example, students preparing for a career in mental health services—and those in in-service training—for example, paraprofessionals and professionals who must learn recently developed evidence-

based approaches to update their practices. In terms of preservice training, university-based curriculum programs have identified a variety of competencies needed for contemporary positions (50–52). Innovators in this area who are training future behavior technicians prefer to target discrete skills rather than overwhelming students with the breadth of facts and principles that constitute the body of knowledge related to mental health. Follow-up research has shown that students who complete these curricula actually pursue careers in their discipline and report that they were adequately prepared for their jobs (52).

A larger body of research has examined the impact of in-service training on the day-to-day practices of mental health treatment providers. Like preservice education, in-service programs for line-level staff have focused on teaching discrete skills that make up the evidence-based practice (53, 54). Trainers use such learning activities as modeling, role play, feedback, and homework to help staff learn new skills and apply them in their treatment settings. Frequently these programs are paired with education for staff on how to use manual-based practices.

Research has shown that service providers who complete these kinds of training programs have improved attitudes about innovative practices (55–60), learn more skills (61–63), and show some use of the skills at their practice setting (33,44,45,62). Skills learned in in-service training are likely to be maintained over time when training is paired with ongoing, regular consultation (16,64,65).

Although education-based approaches are a necessary first step in disseminating evidence-based practices, they have two significant limitations. First, many professionals and paraprofessionals decide not to participate in staff education programs or drop out before training is completed (54,65,66). As a result, a significant portion of the provider population never receives training. Second, treatment providers who learn new skills during in-service training fail to develop enduring treatment services based on these skills (44,49).

In an attempt to identify factors that promote technology transfer, researchers have compared programs that seem to embrace innovative ideas with those that remain stuck in old ways and hence fail to benefit from education approaches (49). They found that in the first case, "innovators" within the program had sufficient organizational commitment and administrative support to introduce and maintain innovations within their teams. Industrial and organizational psychologists have developed a variety of strategies to foster this kind of commitment and support. Some of these strategies are reviewed below.

Education programs are more successful when the use of new skills by staff members is reinforced. Organizational behavior management is the application of behavior modification principles to reinforce individual and group behaviors within organizations (67–69). For example, organizational consultants may teach supervisors and staff how to use work-related rewards, such as extra days off, monetary bonuses, and prime parking spaces, to increase the use of newly learned skills. Organizational behavior management, which is based on B. F. Skinner's form of applied behavior analysis, yields several benefits as a dissemination strategy.

First, it provides the staff developer with a broad and empirically well-supported theoretical perspective for understanding staff behaviors. Professionals who are familiar with behavior modification can quickly master the fundamentals of the strategy (70). Second, this theoretical perspective provides a useful method for tracking the effects of organizational behavior management as well as a useful "bag of tricks" from which training consultants might select such interventions as goal setting (71) and performance feedback (72) to effect desired staff behavior.

Improving
organizational dynamics
A team of treatment providers may not be interacting cohesively for several reasons, as outlined above. Each of these reasons suggests necessary foci for organization-based strategies. Research conducted by organization-al psychologists and management experts from the business sector points to some of these strategies.

Improving team leadership. Research has identified two types of leadership skills that are especially effective for the services team: transformational and transactional (73,74). Leaders who use transformational skills encourage team members to view their work from more elevated perspectives and to develop innovative ways to deal with work-related problems. Specific skills related to transformational leadership promote inspiration, intellectual stimulation, and individual consideration. Transactional leadership skills include goal setting, feedback, self-monitoring, and reinforcement strategies that help team members maintain effective programs.

Two studies have examined whether leadership models that were primarily developed in business and military settings are relevant for mental health and rehabilitation teams (75, 76). Because the goals and tasks that define mental health settings are different from those in industrial and military systems, one might expect that the leadership needs of mental health teams would not be explained by investigations conducted in those systems. However, the research does not support this concern. Findings from studies of more than 1,000 staff members working in human service settings showed that independent groups of mental health providers (77) and rehabilitation providers (76) identified leadership factors that paralleled transformational and transactional leadership. Findings from these studies were then discussed with eight focus groups comprising team members and leaders to develop a curriculum for mental health team leaders (77). Subsequent research found that team leaders who participated in training in this curriculum showed significant improvement in individualized consideration and supervisory feedback (78). Improved leadership has also been associated with consumer satisfaction and quality of life (78).

Total quality management. Targeting leadership skills may often be insufficient to improve teamwork and collaboration. Organizational psychologists have developed total quality management strategies that are useful for facilitating a team's ability to work together and implement effective intervention programs (79–82). Three principles are central to total quality management. First, total quality management is a set of organizational development strategies that attempts to improve the quality and productivity of the work environment from the bottom up—for example, from the level of the case manager, the job coach, and the rehabilitation counselor charged with the day-to-day implementation of the program. Supervisors and administrators are frequently removed from day-to-day affairs and therefore are not aware of immediate programmatic needs (83–85).

Second, development efforts need to be driven by data rather than by opinion (86,87). Hence employees need to collect objective information to identify program needs and client progress. Employees must also collect data to assess the impact of any program development. Finally, total quality management values continuous quality improvement. Staff members are therefore required to make explicit decisions about the program that will improve the quality and productivity of the work environment over time.

Organizational decision-making efforts, such as those supported by total quality management, often fall short when they are general and not specific to the needs of the staff or when they are not conducted for a significant length of time (88–90). Therefore, total quality management efforts that seek to increase evidence-based approaches need to focus specifically on composite skills for an extended period. Few studies of this management style have addressed evidence-based mental health practices, although there has been some study of efforts that affected charting and data-gathering activity in service settings (91,92).

Interactive staff training. Interactive staff training represents an integration of the education approach and the total quality management approach to dissemination (93). As such, it varies from more traditional training efforts in two important ways. First, training focuses on the team in its practice setting; in this way, team members can work together to learn new practices and form them into a viable plan for their agency. Second, it encourages the development of user-friendly programs. Interactive staff training accomplishes these goals by walking the team through four stages.

Stage 1 provides an introduction to the system. Consultants who provide interactive staff training usually come from outside the team. Hence they need to gain the trust of team members before significant training and program development occurs (94). This trust can often be obtained by beginning the training effort with a needs assessment; the message here is that the team best knows its own training needs. Individuals from within the existing team are then assembled as a program committee charged with making preliminary decisions about how to implement the selected intervention. One person from the committee is chosen to champion the training and development effort (21).

In stage 2 a program is developed. Interactive staff training consultants work with the program champion and committee to make specific decisions about which evidence-based practice best meets their needs. The training consultant uses this opportunity to educate committee members and other key staff about the principles and services of the selected intervention. The consultant then engages the program committee in making decisions about how the ideal program will be adapted to meet the needs of participants and staff. Consultants use their expertise to help the committee evaluate initial decisions. Socratic questioning is a useful means for accomplishing this goal (95). Rather than trying to ascertain a weakness or a limitation of a program, the purpose of Socratic questioning is to help the champion and the program committee evaluate for themselves the costs and benefits of specific program choices.

Stage 3 focuses on program implementation. Before a full-fledged trial of the program occurs, the committee pilots a draft program to uncover po-

tential weaknesses. Pilot programs are conducted with a subgroup of team members and a subset of program participants. The program committee then uses a problem-solving approach to resolve difficulties discovered in the pilot program. Through this process, program committees and treatment teams are taught that limitations in an evidenced-based program are problems that can be fixed, rather than overwhelming difficulties that indicate that the program should be abandoned.

Stage 4 covers program maintenance. In the final stage, the team sets up structures that help maintain the newly developed package over the long term. Staff members are en-

▰

There is

a meta-message

in this paper, namely,

that we need to adopt

an evidence-based

approach to evaluating

the dissemination of

evidence-based

treaments.

▰

couraged to brainstorm to produce questions about the efficacy of the program that lead to suggestions for correcting problems. The program committee then collects data to determine program efficacy in terms of the specific questions (96,97). The committee uses the data to adjust the program where needed.

Three studies have examined the impact of interactive staff training on participating staff and their clients. The first study evaluated the impact of nine months of interactive staff training on attitudes and burnout levels of 35 participating staff members

(98). The results showed significant reductions in burnout and improvements in collegial support and in attitudes about program development.

The second study used a team level of analysis to examine whether interactive staff training led to actual change in the behavior of staff who were conducting a rehabilitation program in a residential setting (93). The results showed increases in staff participation in evidence-based services from zero to more than 75 percent of team members. Moreover, the proportion of consumers who participated in targeted strategies rose from less than 10 percent to more than 85 percent of program participants.

The third study obtained similar results with a time series design that measured changes in staff behavior related to the evidence-based program and consumers' response to that program (93). In that study, burnout diminished among all team members. The staff's attitudes about innovations and the actual implementation of the innovations improved significantly. Consumer satisfaction with the program improved, and overall consumer outcome, as measured with the Global Assessment of Functioning, showed significant improvement.

Limitations to research on dissemination programs

There is a meta-message in this paper, namely, that we need to adopt an evidence-based approach to evaluating the dissemination of evidence-based treatments. Although some of the strategies used to evaluate clinical services might be relevant for evaluating dissemination practices, a paradigm for the complete evaluation of transfer strategies would not have the same basic assumptions as one for clinical research (42,93).

Dissemination researchers agree that the comprehensive assessment of training efforts must include five progressively important levels of measurement (99): Did staff participants find the training program interesting and satisfactory? Did training increase the staff's knowledge and skills? Did increased knowledge and skills lead to real changes in the service program? Did consumers report greater satisfaction with the program as a result of these changes? Were consumers better able to cope with their disabilities as a result of program changes?

Much of the dissemination research reviewed in this paper targets the first levels of impact without determining whether staff practices or consumer outcomes actually improve after the dissemination effort.

The standard design for outcomes evaluation in clinical and services research is the randomized controlled trial. However, two obstacles interfere with randomization in dissemination research. First, administrative rules—including union contracts—may prevent the assignment of staff to conditions that represent independent arms of a dissemination impact study. In cases in which such assignments are condoned, administrators might restrict the breadth and depth of process and outcome measures so as not to interfere with work. However, similar concerns are periodically raised as reasons to constrain randomized controlled trials in clinical and service settings. These limitations have been overcome when administrators and policy makers have recognized the importance of this kind of research design.

Second, the rationale behind randomization requires individual service providers to be assigned to different service teams, corresponding with unique dissemination strategies. However, the unit of interest in dissemination research may be the impact of a specific dissemination strategy on the service team; for example, does a specific educational approach improve the assertive community treatment team's ability to provide case management services? Randomly assigning treatment providers to different teams would be like randomly assigning relatives to different families. The size of a randomized trial changes exponentially when the unit of analysis is shifted from individual providers to treatment teams. A study with 60 case managers randomly assigned to a dissemination strategy may have adequate statistical power, but a sample of 60 teams would require many hundred staff in several institutions.

Industrial and organizational psychologists—for example Dansereau and colleagues (100)—have developed research strategies that address this sampling problem. Moreover, quasi-experimental research methods, such as the time series design, or single-subject design methods, such as the multiple-baseline approach, may have to be considered more thoroughly for staff dissemination research.

Evidence-based practices offer great promise for helping people who have serious mental illnesses accomplish their life goals. Some of the staff dissemination practices outlined in this paper will enable service providers in real-life programs to help clients in their efforts. Ongoing research to address the concerns outlined here will ensure that mental health systems use evidence-based dissemination strategies to guide the transfer of effective practices into the practice world. ♦

Acknowledgments

This paper was made possible in part by a grant from the Illinois Office of Mental Health to establish the Illinois Staff Training Institute for Psychiatric Rehabilitation at the University of Chicago.

References

1. Bond G, Becker D, Drake R, et al: Implementing supported employment as an evidence-based practice. Psychiatric Services 52:313–322, 2001

2. Drake RE, Essock SM, Shaner A, et al: Implementing dual diagnosis services for clients with severe mental illness. Psychiatric Services 52:469–476, 2001

3. Phillip SD, Burns BJ, Edgar EJ, et al: Moving assertive community treatment into standard practice. Psychiatric Services 52:771–780, 2001

4. Mellman T, Miller A, Weissman E, et al: Evidence-based pharmacologic treatment for people with severe mental illness: a focus on guidelines and algorithms. Psychiatric Services 52:619–625, 2001

5. Rosenberg SD, Mueser KT, Friedman MJ, et al: Developing effective treatments for posttraumatic disorders among people with severe mental illness. Psychiatric Services 52:1453–1461, 2001

6. Dixon L, McFarlane WR, Lefley H, et al: Evidence-based practices for services to families of people with psychiatric disabilities. Psychiatric Services 52:903–911, 2001

7. Kuipers E: Psychological treatments for psychosis: evidence-based but unavailable? Psychiatric Rehabilitation Skills 4:249–258, 2000

8. Steiner L: Psychiatric rehabilitation in the state mental health system. Psychiatric Rehabilitation Skills (special issue), in press

9. Blair CE, Eldridge EF: An instrument for measuring staff's knowledge of behavior management principles (KBMQ) as applied to geropsychiatric clients in long-term care settings. Journal of Behavior Therapy and Experimental Psychiatry 28:213–220, 1997

10. Dipboye R: Organizational barriers to implementing a rational model of training, in Training for a Rapidly Changing Workplace: Applications of Psychological Research. Edited by Quinones MA, Ehrenstein A. Washington, DC, American Psychological Association, 1997

11. Giffort D: A systems approach to developing staff training. New Directions for Mental Health Services, no 79:25–34, 1998

12. Jonikas J: Staff competencies for service delivery staff in psychosocial rehabilitation programs: a review of the literature. Unpublished manuscript, 1994

13. Torrey W, Bebout R, Kline J, et al: Practice guidelines for clinicians working in programs providing integrated vocational and clinical services for persons with severe mental disorder. Psychiatric Rehabilitation Journal 2:388–393, 1998

14. Haddow M, Milne D: Attributes to community care: development of a questionnaire for professionals. Journal of Mental Health 4:289–296, 1995

15. Good T, Berenbaum H, Nisenson L: Residential caregiver attitudes toward seriously mentally ill persons. Psychiatry 63:23–33, 2000

16. McFarlane WR, McNary S, Dixon L, et al: Predictors of dissemination of family psychoeducation in community mental health centers in Maine and Illinois. Psychiatric Services 52:935–942, 2001

17. Jahr E: Current issues in staff training. Research in Developmental Disabilities 19:73–87, 1998

18. Bernstein G: Training behavior change agents: a conceptual review. Behavior Therapy 13:1–23, 1982

19. Onyett S: Understanding relationships in context as a core competence for psychiatric rehabilitation. Psychiatric Rehabilitation Skills 4:282–299, 2000

20. Rapp C, Wintersteen R: The strengths model of case management: results from twelve demonstrations. Psychosocial Rehabilitation Journal 13(2):23–32, 1989

21. Corrigan PW: Wanted: champions of rehabilitation for psychiatric hospitals. American Psychologist 50:514–521, 1995

22. Corrigan PW, Hess L, Garman AN: Results of a job analysis of psychologists working in state hospitals. Journal of Clinical Psychology 54:1–8, 1998

23. Mueser K, Berenbaum H: Psychodynamic treatment of schizophrenia: is there a future? Psychological Medicine 20:253–262, 1990

24. Dickerson F: Hospital structure and professionals roles, in Handbook of Behavior Therapy in the Psychiatric Setting. Edited by Bellack AS, Hersen M. New York, Plenum, 1993

25. Swiezy N, Matson J: Coordinating the treatment process among various disciplines: behavior analysis and treatment, in Applied Clinical Psychology. Pacific Grove, Calif, Brooks/Cole, 1993

26. Hersen M, Bellack A, Harris F: Staff training and consultation, in Handbook of Behavior Therapy in the Psychiatric Setting. Edited by Bellack AS, Hersen M. New York, Plenum, 1993

27. Silverstein SM, Bowman J, McDugh D: Strategies for hospital-wide dissemination of psychiatric rehabilitation interventions. Psychiatric Rehabilitation Skills 2:1–24, 1997

28. Maslach C, Jackson S, Leiter M: Maslach Burnout Inventory: third edition, in Evaluating Stress: A Book of Resources. Edited by Zalaquett, CAP, Wood, RD. Lanham, Md, Scarecrow Press, 1997

29. Corrigan PW: Differences between clinical and nursing inpatient staff: implications for training in behavioral rehabilitation. Journal of Behavior Therapy and Experimental Psychiatry 25:311–316, 1994

30. Donat D, McKeegan G: Behavioral knowledge and occupational stress among inpatient psychiatric caregivers. Psychiatric Rehabilitation Journal 21:67–69, 1997

31. Corrigan PW, Holmes EP, Luchins D, et al: Staff burnout in psychiatric hospitals: a cross-legged panel design. Journal of Organizational Behavior 15:65–74, 1994

32. Corrigan PW, Williams OB, McCracken SG, et al: Staff attitudes that impede the implementation of behavioral treatment programs. Behavior Interventions 9:1–12, 1998

33. Milne D, Gorenski O, Westerman C, et al: What does it take to transfer training? Psychiatric Rehabilitation Skills 4:259–281, 2000

34. Walko S, Pratt C, Siiter R, et al: Predicting staff retention in psychiatric rehabilitation. Psychosocial Rehabilitation Journal 16(3):150–153, 1993

35. Reid D, Everson J, Green C: A systematic evaluation of preferences identified through person-centered planning for people with profound multiple disabilities. Journal of Applied Behavior Analysis 32:467–477, 1999

36. Corrigan PW, Kwartarini WY, Pramana W: Staff perceptions of barriers to behavior therapy in a psychiatric hospital. Behavior Modification 16:132–144, 1992

37. Bass B: From transactional to transformational leadership: learning to share the vision. Organizational Dynamics 18:19–31, 1990

38. Howell J, Hall-Merenda K: The ties that bind: the impact of leader-member exchange, transformational and transactional leadership, and distance on predicting follower performance. Journal of Applied Psychology 84:680–694, 1999

39. Sosik J, Dionne S: Leadership styles and Deming's behavior factors. Journal of Business and Psychology 11:447–462, 1997

40. Barlow DH: On the relation of clinical research to clinical practice: current issues, new directions. Journal of Consulting and Clinical Psychology 49:147–155, 1981

41. Addis M, Wade W, Hatgis C: Barriers to dissemination of evidence-based practices: addressing practitioners' concerns about manual-based psychotherapies. Clinical Psychology 6:430–441, 1999

42. Anthony W: Psychiatric rehabilitation technology: operationalizing the "black box" of the psychiatric rehabilitation process. New Directions for Mental Health Services, no 79:79–87, 1998

43. Eckman T, Liberman R, Phipps C, et al: Teaching medication management skills to schizophrenic patients. Journal of Clinical Psychopharmacology 10:33–38, 1990

44. Wallace CJ, Liberman RP, MacKain SJ, et al: Effectiveness and replicability of modules for teaching social and instrumental skills to the severely mentally ill. American Journal of Psychiatry 149:654–658, 1992

45. Kavanagh DJ, Piatkowska O, Clark D, et al: Application of cognitive behavioral interventions for schizophrenia in multidisciplinary teams: what can the matter be? Australian Psychologist 28:181–188, 1993

46. Drake R, Becker D, Clark P, et al: Research on the individual placement and support model of supported employment. Psychiatric Quarterly 70(4):289–301, 1999

47. Cohen M, Farkas M, Nemec P: Psychiatric rehabilitation programs: putting concepts into practice? Community Mental Health Journal 24:7–21, 1988

48. Test MA, Stein L: Practical guidelines for the community treatment of markedly impaired patients. Community Mental Health Journal 36:47–60, 2000

49. Corrigan PW, MacKain SJ, Liberman RP: Skills training modules: a strategy for dissemination and utilization of a rehabilitation innovation, in Intervention Research. Edited by Rothman J, Thomas E. Chicago, Haworth, 1994

50. Anthony W, Cohen M, Farkas M, et al: The chronically mentally ill case management: more than a response to a dysfunctional system. Community Mental Health Journal 24:219–228, 1988

51. Backs AB, Giffort DW, McCracken SG, et al: Public academic training partnership for paraprofessionals who provide psychiatric rehabilitation. Psychiatric Rehabilitation Skills, in press

52. Gill KJ, Pratt CW, Barrett N: Preparing psychiatric rehabilitation specialists through undergraduate education. Community Mental Health Journal 33:323–329, 1997

53. Pratt C, Gill K: Profit sharing in psychiatric rehabilitation: a five-year evaluation. Psychosocial Rehabilitation Journal 17(2):33–41, 1993

54. Rogers ES, Cohen BF, Danley KS, et al: Training mental health workers in psychiatric rehabilitation. Schizophrenia Bulletin 12:709–719, 1986

55. Addleton R, Tratnack S, Donat D: Hospital-based multidisciplinary training in the care of seriously mentally ill patients. Hospital and Community Psychiatry 42:60–61, 1991

56. Barnett JE, Clendenen F: The quality journey in a comprehensive mental health center. JCAHO Journal on Quality Improvement 22:8–17, 1996

57. Berryman J, Evans IM, Kalbag A: The effects of training in nonaversive behavior management on the attitudes and understanding of direct care staff. Journal of Behavior Therapy and Experimental Psychiatry 25:241–250, 1994

58. Cook J, Yamaguchi J, Solomon M: Field-testing a post-secondary faculty in-service training for working with students who have psychiatric disabilities. Psychosocial Rehabilitation Journal 17(2):157–170, 1993

59. Liberman RP, Eckman T: Dissemination of skills training modules to psychiatric facilities: overcoming obstacles to the utilisation of a rehabilitation innovation. British Journal of Psychiatry 155(suppl 5):117–122, 1989

60. Lam C, Chan F, Hillburger J: Canonical relationships between vocational interests and attitudes. Vocational Evaluation and Work Adjustment Bulletin 26:155–160, 1993

61. Cook J, Horton-O'Connell T, Fitzgibbon G, et al: Training for state-funded providers of assertive community treatment. New Directions for Mental Health Services, no 79:55–64, 1998

62. Fadden G: Implementation of family interventions in routine clinical practice following staff training programs: a major cause for concern. Journal of Mental Health (UK) 6:599–612, 1997

63. Rubel E, Sobell L, Miller W: Do continuing education workshops improve participants' skills? Effects of a motivational interviewing workshop on substance abuse counselors' skills and knowledge. AABT Behavior Therapist (Association for Advancement of Behavior Therapy) 23:73–80, 2000

64. Donat D: Impact of a mandatory behavioral consultation on seclusion/restraint utilization in a psychiatric hospital. Journal of Behavior Therapy and Experimental Psychiatry 29:13–19, 1998

65. Liberman RP, Eckman T, Kuehnel T, et al: Dissemination of new behavior therapy programs to community mental health programs. American Journal of Psychiatry 139:224–226, 1982

66. Liberman RP, Nuechterlein K, Wallace C: Social skills training and the nature of schizophrenia, in Social Skills Training: A Practical Handbook for Assessment and Treatment. Edited by Curran JP, Monti PM. New York, New York University Press, 1986

67. Bucklin B, Alvero A, Dickinson A, et al: Industrial-organizational psychology and organizational behavior management: an ob-

jective comparison. Journal of Organizational Behavior Management 20:27–75, 2000

68. Frederiksen L: Handbook of Organizational Behavior Management. New York, Wiley, 1982

69. Reid D, Parsons M: Organizational behavior management in human service settings, in Handbook of Applied Behavior Analysis. Edited by Austin J, Carr JE. Reno, Nev, Context Press, 2000

70. Milne D: Organizational behavior management in a psychiatric day hospital. Behavioral Psychotherapy 16:177–188, 1988

71. Calpin J, Edelstein B, Redmon W: Performance feedback and goal setting to improve mental health center staff productivity. Journal of Organizational Behavior Management 9:35–58, 1988

72. Green C, Reid D, Perkins L, et al: Increasing habilitative services for persons with profound handicaps: an application of structural analysis to staff management. Journal of Applied Behavior Analysis 24:459–471, 1991

73. Avolio B, Bass B, Jung D: Re-examining the components of transformational and transactional leadership using the multifactor leadership questionnaire. Journal of Occupational and Organizational Psychiatry 72:441–462, 1999

74. Bass B: Current developments in transformational leadership: research and applications. Psychologist-Manager Journal 3(1):5–21, 1999

75. Corrigan PW, Garman AN, Lam C, et al: What mental health teams want in their leaders. Administration and Policy in Mental Health 26:111–124, 1998

76. Corrigan PW, Garman AN, Canar J, et al: Characteristics of rehabilitation team leaders: a validation study. Rehabilitation Counseling Bulletin 42:186–195, 1999

77. Garman AN, Corrigan PW: Developing effective team leaders. New Directions for Mental Health Services, no 79:45–54, 1998

78. Corrigan PW, Lickey SE, Campion J, et al: A short course in leadership skills for the rehabilitation team. Journal of Rehabilitation 66:56–58, 2000

79. Deming WE: Out of Crisis. Cambridge, Mass, Institute of Technology Center for Advanced Engineering Study, 1986

80. Victor B, Boynton A, Stephens-Jahng T: The effective design of work under total quality management. Organizational Science 2:102–117, 2000

81. Priebe S: Ensuring and improving quality in community mental health care. International Review of Psychiatry 12:226–232, 2000

82. Sluyter G: Total quality management in behavioral health care. New Directions for Mental Health Services, no 79:35–43, 1998

83. Marks ML, Mirvis P, Hackett E, et al: Employee participation in a quality circle program: impact on quality of work life, productivity, and absenteeism. Journal of Applied Psychology 71:61–69, 1986

84. Yeager E: Examining the quality control circle. Personnel Journal 58:682–708, 1979

85. Zemke R: Honeywell imports quality circles as long-term management strategy. Training 17:6–10, 1980

86. Barter JT, Lall K: Accreditation, in Textbook of Administrative Psychiatry. Edited by Talbott JA, Hales RE, Keill SL. Washington, DC, American Psychiatric Press, 1992

87. Fauman M: Quality assurance monitoring, in Manual of Psychiatric Quality Assurance. Edited by Mattson, MR. Washington, DC, American Psychiatric Association, 1992

88. Bowditch JL, Buono AF: A Primer on Organizational Behavior, 3rd ed. New York, Wiley, 1994

89. Glaser EM, Backer TE: Organization development in mental health services. Administration in Mental Health 6:195–215, 1979

90. Pearlstein R: Who empowers leaders? Performance Improvement Quarterly 4(4):12–20, 1991

91. Hunter ME, Love CC: Total quality management and the reduction of inpatient violence and costs in a forensic psychiatric hospital. Psychiatric Services 47:751–754, 1996

92. Sluyter GV, Mukherjee AK: Total Quality Management for Mental Health and Mental Retardation Services: A Paradigm for the '90s. Annandale, Va, American Network of Community Options and Resources, 1993

93. Corrigan PW, McCracken SG: An interactive approach to training teams and developing programs. New Directions for Mental Health Services, no 79:3–12, 1998

94. Brooker C, Tarrier N, Barrowclough C: Training community psychiatric nurses for psychosocial intervention. British Journal of Psychiatry 160:836–844, 1992

95. Griffith B, Frieden G: Facilitating reflective thinking in counselor education. Counselor Education and Supervision 40:82–93, 2000

96. Bickman L, Noser K: Meeting the challenges in the delivery of child and adolescent mental health services in the next millennium: the continuous quality improvement approach. Applied and Preventive Psychology 8:247–255, 1999

97. Wandersman A, Imm P, Chinman M, et al: Getting to outcomes: a results-based approach to accountability. Evaluation and Program Planning 23:389–395, 2000

98. Corrigan PW, Holmes EP, Luchins D, et al: The effects of interactive staff training on staff programming and patient aggression in a psychiatric unit. Behavioral Interventions 10:17–32, 1995

99. Thomas EJ, Rothman J: Intervention Research: Design and Development for Human Service. New York, Haworth, 1994

100. Dansereau F, Yammarino F, Kohles J: Multiple levels of analysis from a longitudinal perspective: some implications for theory building. Academy of Management Review 24:346–357, 1999

Integrating Evidence-Based Practices and the Recovery Model

Frederick J. Frese III, Ph.D.
Jonathan Stanley, J.D.
Ken Kress, J.D., Ph.D.
Suzanne Vogel-Scibilia, M.D.

Consumer advocacy has emerged as an important factor in mental health policy during the past few decades. Winning consumer support for evidence-based practices requires recognition that consumers' desires and needs for various types of treatments and services differ significantly. The authors suggest that the degree of support for evidence-based practices by consumer advocates depends largely on the degree of disability of the persons for whom they are advocating. Advocates such as members of the National Alliance for the Mentally Ill, who focus on the needs of the most seriously disabled consumers, are most likely to be highly supportive of research that is grounded in evidence-based practices. On the other hand, advocates who focus more on the needs of consumers who are further along their road to recovery are more likely to be attracted to the recovery model. Garnering the support of this latter group entails ensuring that consumers, as they recover, are given increasing autonomy and greater input about the types of treatments and services they receive. The authors suggest ways to integrate evidence-based practices with the recovery model and then suggest a hybrid theory that maximizes the virtues and minimizes the weaknesses of each model.

Shortly after the National Institute of Mental Health was returned to the National Institutes of Health in 1989, President George H. W. Bush declared the "Decade of the Brain." Federal funding for research on the brain was greatly increased during that time, resulting in remarkable scientific progress (1). The 1990s saw advances not only in our understanding of the working of the human brain but also in our approaches to the treatment of the mental illnesses that are caused by brain abnormalities. During the past decade, confidence in scientific research, with its objective observations and measures, has increased considerably in the mental health arena.

Evidence-based practices

In recent years, this increased confidence in scientific treatment methods for mental illnesses has given rise to a movement that calls for more widespread adoption of treatment approaches that are scientifically grounded. This movement has been developing under the rubric of "evidence-based practices" (2–7). Under this concept, the call for greater reliance on scientific evidence is being extended to treatment approaches that are supported by psychological and sociological evidence as well as by the findings of biological research.

In an earlier article on evidence-based practices, Drake and associates (3) provided an overview of the topic, outlining the research findings and philosophical underpinnings of the evidence-based practice movement. They spelled out specific reasons for the special focus by *Psychiatric Services* on evidence-based practice interventions. These reasons include the belief that routine mental health programs do not provide evidence-based practices, that implementation of services resembling evidence-based practices may lack fidelity to evidence-based procedures, and, especially, that in the context of limited resources consumers have a right to interventions that are known to be effective. So described, evidence-based practices appear to be unassailable. Who could object to promoting the use of treatments that work rather than those that do not?

Drake and colleagues (3) also delineated a core set of interventions: prescription of medications within specific parameters, training in self-management of illness, assertive community treatment, family psychoeducation, supported employment, and integrated treatment for co-occurring substance use disorders. The authors stressed that "mental health services for persons with severe mental illness

Dr. Frese is assistant professor of psychology in clinical psychiatry at the Northeastern Ohio Universities College of Medicine and former first vice-president of the National Alliance for the Mentally Ill (NAMI). Mr. Stanley is assistant director of the Treatment Advocacy Center in Arlington, Virginia. Dr. Kress is professor of law and director of the Mental Health Law Project at the University of Iowa College of Law in Iowa City. Dr. Vogel-Scibilia is a psychiatrist in private practice in Beaver, Pennsylvania, and a board member of NAMI. All of the authors are active consumer advocates. Send correspondence to Dr. Frese at the Recovery Project, c/o ADM Board, 100 West Cedar Street, Suite 300, Akron, Ohio 44307 (e-mail, fjfrese@infi.net). This article was originally published in the November 2001 issue of Psychiatric Services.

should reflect the goals of consumers."

Drake and colleagues further stated that "mental health services should not focus exclusively on traditional outcomes such as compliance with treatment and relapse or rehospitalization prevention, but should be broadened to include helping people to attain such consumer-oriented outcomes as: independence, employment, satisfying relationships, and good quality of life." Finally, they allowed that evidence-based practices "do not provide the answers for all persons with mental illness, all outcomes, or all settings" (3).

In light of this characterization of evidence-based practices, particularly the openness to consumers' needs and aspirations, one might expect that the consumer advocacy community would be pleased that the views of consumers are emerging as a major matter of interest. This move beyond traditional, "provider-centric" factors seems to be a healthy, consumer-friendly development. In consumer advocacy circles, "Nothing about us without us" has increasingly been adopted as a slogan for expressing the desire for more dignity and autonomous control for the recipients of mental health services (8). This reaching out for consumer input should be a welcome development.

The recovery model
At the same time that the Decade of the Brain initiatives and evidence-based initiatives have been emerging in the mental health arena, a more personalized and subjective approach to caring for persons who have mental illness has also been emerging—the recovery model.

William Anthony, a major supporter of the recovery model (9), describes recovery as "a deeply personal, unique process of changing one's attitudes, values, feelings, goals, skills, and/or roles. It is a way of living a satisfying, hopeful, and contributing life, even with limitations caused by the illness. Recovery involves the development of new meaning and purpose in one's life as one grows beyond the catastrophic effects of mental illness." Sullivan (10) called for "a broad definition of recovery, one that not only focuses on the management of the ill-

ness, but also highlights the consumer's performance of instrumental role functions and notions of empowerment and self-directedness."

The recovery model emphasizes that responsibility for and control of the recovery process must be given in large part to the person who has the condition. Indeed, some advocates for the recovery model have stressed that overdependence on others prevents recovery. The locus of control thus becomes less external. Mental health interventions are designed to be empowering, enabling the persons themselves to take responsibility for decisions about their lives (11,12). Recently, some states—for example, Wisconsin and Ohio—have been redesigning their mental health systems to stress recovery-model values, such as hope, healing, empowerment, social connectedness, human rights, and recovery-oriented services (12).

Although the recovery model has been garnering support among consumer advocates and mental health administrators, objections to this approach have recently been raised among mental health professionals. Pointing out that the recovery model is subjective, not data based or scientific, Peyser (13) suggested that it may in fact interfere with treatment. He pointed out that psychotic illnesses and similar illnesses can subvert the thinking process to the point that the patient's self is taken over by the disease. He asked how we can speak about empowerment and collaboration in such cases and suggested that there are "dangers in going too far" toward fashioning a model that focuses primarily on hope, empowerment, and human rights.

Two apparently very different approaches to treatment of mentally ill persons are emerging. The scientific, objective, evidence-based approach emphasizes external scientific reality, whereas the recovery model stresses the importance of the phenomenological, subjective experiences and autonomous rights of persons who are in recovery. The two models will conflict under many circumstances. Obviously, when consumers make decisions about treatment, they will sometimes make choices that are not evidence based. Treatment decisions

cannot be made entirely on factual, scientific grounds. Rather, treatment decisions involve both medical facts and choices based on values.

Science can identify alternative possible treatments and an outcome-probability distribution of efficacy and adverse effects for each treatment option. The decision as to which combination of anticipated improvement and anticipated adverse effects is preferable is a value judgment. Consumers' decisions about treatment will be more likely to reflect their values than will decisions by treating professionals, even when professionals attempt to determine consumers' preferences. Thus evidence-based treatments may differ from treatments that are based on the recovery model insofar as they reflect different judgments of the value of various treatment outcomes by service providers and consumers.

The recovery model has found significant support in the mental health field, particularly among consumer advocates. Thus the question arises as to whether these apparently opposed approaches to mental health care can coexist. And can efforts to expand the influence of evidence-based practices somehow accommodate the more subjective philosophical thrust of the recovery movement?

Increasing the use of externally derived interventions while maximizing individual empowerment that emanates from an internal locus of control will be a challenge. However, if we are to win consumer advocacy support for evidence-based practices, we should accommodate the insights of the recovery movement.

Integrating the recovery model and evidence-based practices ·
One approach to reconciling scientific and subjective approaches to treatment was recently suggested by Munetz and Frese (14). They suggested that the traditional evidence-based approach—the "medical model"—can be compatible with the recovery model. In their view, the evidence-based, medical model has been highly paternalistic, emphasizing illness, weakness, and limitations rather than the potential for growth. They claimed that the evidence-

based medical model has been perceived as stamping out hope by implying that biology is destiny and emphasizing an external locus of control. They also mentioned that some consumer advocates view the physician as a powerful and oppressive figure who "at best is acting out of misguided beneficence" and at worst fosters "helplessness and chronicity."

Munetz and Frese also described extreme critics of the medical model who accept Szasz's position that mental illnesses do not really exist as biopsychosocial disorders (15). However, they also pointed out that some consumer advocates, including the psychologists Deegan (16,17) and Frese (18,19), accept the existence of their illnesses and recognize that they have certain limitations because of their illness. Deegan (17), however, also warned of the "cycle of disempowerment and despair" that is engendered by traditional, objectively based, paternalistic approaches to treatment of mentally ill persons.

Munetz and Frese (14) have shown how this alleged conflict between objectivity and subjectivity can be largely resolved. For persons who are so seriously impaired in their decision-making capacity that they are incapable of determining what is in their best interest, a paternalistic, externally reasoned treatment approach seems not only appropriate but also necessary in most cases for the well-being of the impaired individual. However, as these impaired persons begin to benefit from externally initiated interventions, the locus of control should increasingly shift from the treatment provider to the person who is recovering. As individuals recover, they must gradually be afforded a larger role in the selection of treatments and services. Throughout the recovery process, persons should be given maximal opportunity to regain control over their lives. They should be given increasingly greater choice about evidence-based interventions and other available services.

To accommodate the precepts of the evidence-based medical model with those of the recovery model, Munetz and Frese suggested an approach consonant with the observations of Csernansky and Bardgett and others. After surveying recent research on the pathophysiology of the brain, Csernansky and Bardgett (20) pointed out that the degree of impairment in serious mental illnesses falls somewhere on a continuum that ranges from severe, refractory psychosis to less serious, responsive psychosis and on toward normality.

Munetz and Frese (14) pointed out that many individuals are so disabled with mental illness that they do not have the capacity to understand that they are ill. Giving such individuals the right to make decisions about their treatment is tantamount to abandonment. They noted that it is "inconsistent with the recovery paradigm to allow incapacitated individuals to remain victims of their serious mental illness." For these persons, measures must be taken so that they become well enough to be able to benefit from the recovery model. That is, one treatment goal whose significance should be accentuated by evidence-based practices is enhancement of the consumer's ability to make autonomous decisions about treatment as a means of gaining control of his or her treatment.

Thus persons who are very disabled by mental illness are those most likely to benefit from objective, evidence-based approaches to treatment. For these persons there is less of a need to focus on the person-centered principles of the recovery model. However, as such persons begin to benefit from treatments, they should be afforded opportunity for greater autonomy. As they progress along the road to recovery, their growing capacity for autonomy should be respected, eventually to the point at which treatment personnel assume the role of consultants and virtually all decisions about treatment are in the hands of the persons who are making the journey of recovery.

Persons who have substantially recovered can be viewed as those likely to benefit the most from the autonomy-centered recovery model. Alternatively, such persons could be viewed as having sufficient capacity for autonomy to have the same right to make their own decisions about treatment—even if those decisions are not evidence based or maximally therapeutic—as is routinely accorded to persons who are viewed as having no decision-making impairments.

Consumers' views

An important and logical step in increasing consumer empowerment is to identify the concerns of the consumer. Attempts to determine how psychiatrically disabled persons perceive their needs is a relatively new concept in mental health. Until the latter part of the 20th century, persons with schizophrenia and other serious mental illnesses were generally viewed as being so delusional or otherwise cognitively impaired that they were incapable of providing substantive input about their care. Although many such persons did recover, the opprobrium they faced was so ingrained that few of them, or even their family members, would openly acknowledge their experiences with these conditions. As is the case today, there were significant disincentives to make such disclosures for those who were, or had been, considered "insane." A similar stigma discouraged openness by persons who had "insanity in the family."

However, beginning in the 1960s, some persons who had been subjected to treatment for serious mental illnesses began to identify themselves openly. In addition, some of these recovering persons took steps to organize themselves and started to give voice to their views. The advocacy efforts of consumers and family members have mushroomed and today represent a valuable and formidable force that affects all aspects of mental health policy (21).

The National Alliance for the Mentally Ill

Of the consumer advocacy entities that were formed during the past quarter century, the National Alliance for the Mentally Ill (NAMI) is by far the largest. NAMI was founded as recently as 1979. As of the summer of 2001, NAMI had a membership of more than 210,000—with more than 1,200 affiliates—located in all 50 states. NAMI currently supports a full-time staff of more than 60.

NAMI initially functioned as a group that advocated primarily for the families of persons with serious mental illnesses. However, the influence of the consumers in NAMI has become increasingly important. The organization has a large consumer council. During the past several years at least one quarter of the members of NAMI's board of directors have been consumers. However, despite this growing influence, the tens of thousands of consumer members of NAMI do not speak as an independent organization but blend their concerns with those of the majority of the NAMI members—for the most part, family members.

NAMI has a long and complex policy agenda but recently has given special prominence to what the organization sees as eight particularly important policy issues. These priorities are characterized by NAMI as being "based on the most effective standards and programs demonstrated to empower individuals on the road to recovery." Published and widely distributed as the "Omnibus Mental Illness Recovery Act: A Blueprint for Recovery—OMIRA" (22), these eight NAMI priorities are participation by consumers and their family members in planning of mental illness services; equitable health care coverage, or parity, in health insurance; access to newer medications; assertive community treatment; work incentives for persons who have severe mental illness; reduction in life-threatening and harmful actions and restraints; reduction in the criminalization of persons who have severe mental illness; and access to permanent, safe, and affordable housing with appropriate community-based services.

There is noticeable overlap between NAMI's policy priorities and the six core interventions outlined by Drake and colleagues. One area—assertive community treatment—is clearly prioritized, under the same term, by both NAMI and proponents of evidence-based practices. The call for prescription of medications within specific parameters is somewhat addressed by NAMI's prioritizing access to newer medications. Moreover, NAMI was an active participant in the public launch of the findings of the Schizophrenia Patient Outcomes Research Team (PORT), which gave wide distribution to the specific rec-

ommended parameters for prescribed antipsychotic medications (23). NAMI also produced and distributed more than 500,00 brochures highlighting these recommendations.

These efforts, which support the PORT results, also highlighted the recommended evidence-based interventions for assertive community treatment and for family psychoeducation. Indeed, although neither is explicitly designated as an evidence-based practice, NAMI has two major training initiatives related to psychoeducation: the Family-to-Family program, which focuses on education of family members, and the Living With Schizophrenia program, which teaches consumers to better live with their disorders. This latter effort primarily involves self-management of illness and thus is also related to another of the designated core interventions of Drake and colleagues.

The fifth core initiative under the evidence-based practice model—supported employment—is encompassed in OMIRA under work incentives for persons with severe mental illness, even though the two are not identical. Finally, although NAMI has yet to develop an explicit policy initiative that calls for integrated mental health and substance abuse treatment, the national NAMI board has been actively weighing the pros and cons of taking a position that supports this initiative.

In a broader yet specific demonstration of support by NAMI for the six evidence-based practice initiatives, the president of the NAMI board recently sent a letter to all 16 national board members that highlighted the importance of the evidence-based practices movement.

NAMI, of course, was started by family members of persons who were very disabled with mental illnesses. The needs of the most disabled persons continues to be the organization's priority. Many of the consumers for whom NAMI lobbies tend to be too disabled to effectively speak for themselves. Many of them are not ready to benefit from the recovery model. NAMI can be expected to provide strong support for evidence-based practice initiatives but will not necessarily be uncritical. On

the other hand, agenda statements have been made by organized groups of consumer advocates during the past decade that have presented the collective voices of persons who are further along in their recovery—persons who are better able to speak for themselves.

The National Mental Health Consumers' Association

One of the more successful attempts to characterize the spectrum of concerns of recovering persons is embodied in the mission statement and the national agenda of the National Mental Health Consumers' Association (NMHCA). Although the organization has not been active during the past few years, from the mid-1980s through the mid-1990s it was widely viewed as the most organized and largest independent, non-disease-specific organization for persons who had been treated for serious mental illness.

Consumer advocates all over the country regularly participated in the election of members of the NMHCA board. Meeting monthly via conference call, the board had some claim to reflecting the collective voice of consumers' concerns nationally because of NMHCA's organizational structure. In the early 1990s and after lengthy deliberations, NMHCA produced a mission statement and a national agenda. The wording of their documents was approved overwhelmingly by both the board and the NMHCA membership in attendance at their meeting held December 12, 1992, in Philadelphia during the annual national Alternatives Conference. Although the NMHCA mission statement was widely distributed in consumer advocacy circles, to our knowledge it has not previously been published.

Examination of NMHCA's mission and national agenda statements (see box) reveals that NMHCA's priorities are, by and large, dissimilar from the evidence-based practice initiatives. Although the latter focus heavily on the use of medications and on other services, NMHCA's priorities primarily stress factors that should better enable recovering persons to more easily integrate into society. Indeed, the six items on NMHCA's national agenda overlap very little with stated targets of the evidence-based practice core interventions. The NMHCA agenda item on benefits calls for entitlement to comprehensive health care. This may or may not include various types of mental health care; such care is explicitly mentioned only in the items on mental health systems and self-help. In addition, the major focus of these latter items is on more consumer-oriented priorities in the overall structure of the mental health system, not on increased availability of psychiatric services.

The statement of NMHCA's priorities is, in essence, a call for a reexamination of the philosophy and focus of the mental health establishment. It endorses the primary purpose of the development and implementation of mental health services to be for "recovery and healing," not for "social control." The individuals constructing and supporting NMHCA's statement of its national priorities are apparently reasonably far along in their own recovery. Indeed, they appear to be sufficiently recovered to focus primarily on how they can reduce environmental barriers to recovery rather than on examining which treatments they should be receiving. NMHCA advocates who are mostly recovered clearly argue for a more internal locus of control.

This heavy stress on increased autonomy and other recovery priorities by consumer advocates who are mostly recovered fits well with an approach that increases the consumer's autonomy as recovery progresses. However, a serious question remains about the degree to which the views of NMHCA activists reflect the concerns of nonactivist consumers who are less recovered and perhaps less articulate. Similarly, some advocates of the recovery model may not reflect the concerns or needs of this latter group of consumers.

To our knowledge, no national attempt has been made to systematically capture the sentiment of consumers who are more seriously disabled. Attempts have been made in several states to survey such consumers about their views on services. One of the more active of these efforts has been under way in Ohio for the past five years or so.

NMHCA mission statement and agenda

Mission statement
Guided by the principles of choice, empowerment, and self-determination, the National Mental Health Consumers' Association is a human rights organization that advocates for employment, housing, benefits, service choice, and the end of discrimination and abuse in the lives of persons who use, have used, or have been used by the mental health systems.

National agenda
Employment. We support the full implementation of the Americans With Disabilities Act and the Rehabilitation Services Act. We must be given every opportunity to be gainfully employed in occupations where we, with reasonable accommodation, can contribute. We call upon the mental health system to practice affirmative action in training and employing mental health consumers in professional careers in the mental health system.

Housing. All persons, particularly those identified as being mentally ill, are entitled to adequate, permanent homes of their choice.

Benefits. All psychiatrically disabled persons must be entitled to sufficient income, social supports, and comprehensive health care to enjoy an adequate quality of life.

Mental health systems. Recovery and healing, not social control, must be the goal and outcome of the mental health system; therefore, the mental health system must be client driven.

Self-help. We support the full and sustained funding and development of user-run alternatives and additions to the traditional mental health system, self-determined and governed by and for members, in every community.

Discrimination. Discrimination, abuse, ostracism, stigmatization, and other forms of social prejudice must be identified and vigorously opposed at every opportunity.

Ohio consumer quality review teams

Beginning in 1996, consumer quality review teams were established by the Ohio Department of Mental Health to determine consumers' views of the mental health delivery system in 22 of Ohio's 88 counties. Although a few family members and professionals participated as employees in the teams' projects, the overwhelming majority of employees were persons in recovery from serious mental illness. The primary method for collecting data about consumers' perceived needs in this team effort was through consumer-conducted, structured individual interviews, each of which lasted for up to two hours.

From July 1996 to March 1999 some 890 adult consumers of Ohio's public services for the seriously mentally ill were individually interviewed about their views of mental health services. Consumers volunteered for participation in the project. Their names were drawn in a quasi-randomized, stratified manner from both rural and urban areas of the state.

An analysis of the data gathered from these Ohio consumers indicated three general areas of concern (24). One was services that consumers believed were needed but either were not available or were seriously undersupplied: crisis stabilization, longer-term secure residential programs, clubhouse services, housing, meaningful retraining and job placement opportunities, and consumer-run services, which were reported to be "highly valued" by consumers.

These consumers, as a group, also indicated that they viewed some services as being both available and particularly helpful. These were emotional support, education and information, social support, treatment, stabilization, and financial support. A third area of consumer interest related to aspects of care that were seen as needing the greatest improvement: access to services, adequate numbers of staff, greater consumer influence, and more considerate behavior from mental health staff. One final finding of note was that a significant proportion of consumers was unsure or unaware of which services were in fact being provided in their areas.

The consumers who were interviewed by the consumer quality review teams were all clients of the public mental health system in Ohio. Attempts were made to ensure a maximally random selection of subjects, so one could conclude that this sample of opinions was more representative of the "typical" person who has serious mental illness than those who structured the NMHCA priorities.

Nevertheless, the consumers stressed several of NMHCA's priorities. These include housing, consumer-run activities, increased consumer influence, benefits such as financial and social support, and access to treatment and health care services. However, unlike the NMHCA advocates who are further recovered, these consumers expressed a desire for services that resembled evidence-based practice interventions. These include the explicit mention of medication, presumably in appropriate dosages; education and information, similar to training in illness self-management and family psychoeducation; retraining and job placement opportunities, which could include supported employment; and more staff as well as staff who are more understanding, both of which are, or should be, components of assertive community treatment.

Thus the findings of the consumer quality review teams suggest that consumers who are probably not as far into their recovery may be more receptive to the types of services that make up the core interventions of the evidence-based practice model. More detailed and current information about the Ohio consumer quality review teams can be found on the Web sites www.qsan.org and www.qrsinc.org.

Discussion and conclusions

Over the past three decades, increasingly influential consumer voices have emerged and have advocated for improvements in the treatment of persons who have mental illness. Two recently developing philosophical forces are competing for the support of these newly enfranchised consumers. One of them is based on science, premised on the identification and implementation of modalities that have been demonstrated by scientific evidence to be effective. The other is the recovery model, which emphasizes the personal nature of the recovery journeys and insists that the final arbiter of how one should recover should be the person who is recovering.

This article has reviewed the viewpoints of three groups of consumers. Although there are numerous similarities, such as a unanimous call for adequate housing, the positions of the various consumer advocates largely reflect the degree of disability of those for whom they are advocating. Those who represent the most disabled, such as family members who believe that they are advocating for those who are not capable of speaking rationally for themselves, tend to be very supportive of evidence-based practice initiatives. Consumers who themselves have recovered fairly well tend to stress the importance of taking control of their own lives. Such persons value their own ability to make choices and even their ability to risk failure. For them, the improvements in treatment that accompany evidence-based practices may be important, but not as important as the rights of consumers to make their own decisions about what services are best for them. As they see it, they themselves—and not more detached scientific researchers—must be the final arbiters of how they will go about their recovery.

Examining the views of consumers who tend to be sufficiently recovered to be able to rationally discuss their opinions, but not so recovered as to have become "advocates," we find the desire for a little of both worlds. These consumers want better treatments, but they also desire more influence and autonomy.

These observations have several implications for those who are interested in garnering maximal support for evidence-based practice initiatives. NAMI members and other advocates who sometimes speak for "those who cannot speak for themselves" are likely to be very receptive to evidence-based practice initiatives. Indeed, the NAMI leadership already has indicated a willingness to help support and implement evidence-based practice interventions. Those who are interested in encouraging consumer advocacy support for evidence-based practices are likely to find significant assistance here.

On the other hand, advocates who speak for consumers who are further along the recovery process often belong to this group of consumers themselves. They tend to be more focused on regaining personal control, placing a higher priority on rights and opportunities to improve quality of life. They also desire more interaction and influence with the groups that make mental health decisions that affect their lives.

To better gain support from these consumer advocates, a number of actions might be considered. First, more consumers can be invited to participate in groups that are responsible for conducting, overseeing, and implementing evidence-based practice activities. As changes to treatments are being considered, having consumers "at the table" goes a long way toward letting them feel that their contributions are valued and that the decision-making process is fair.

Second, because participation in discussions of scientific matters usually requires familiarity with scientific methods and principles, better efforts should be made to encourage graduate and professional schools that train and accredit mental health providers to recruit consumers in recovery. Such efforts could help increase the number of consumers who are able to contribute to the development and implementation of evidence-based practice interventions. Some academic entities, such as the Nova Southeastern University Center for Psychological Studies and the Program in Psychiatric Rehabilitation of the University of Medicine and Dentistry of New Jersey, have made good starts in this direction, but the number of such efforts is woefully small.

Third, a small but growing number of psychiatrists, psychologists, social workers, and other mental health professionals who are in recovery from mental illness have decided to openly identify themselves as such. Psychiatrists Carol North (25), Dan Fisher (26), and Suzanne Vogel-Scibilia (27) have all publicly declared that they have experienced serious mental illness. Psychologists Ronald Bassman (28), Al Siebert (29), Kay Jamison (30), and Wendy Walker Davis (31) and social workers Donna Orrin (32) and David Granger (33) have made similar disclosures. In all probability, many other such professionals are also in recovery. If these professionals could begin to be more open about their experiences and those of their family members, consumer advocates could better realize that mental health policy and research decisions are not being made as much in isolation from consumer influence as it may appear.

Most consumers fall somewhere between the two ends of the cognitive impairment spectrum. These individuals, when asked, appear to desire more control and influence but also seem to realize that they need more and better treatment. In that this is the group that probably constitutes the majority of those served by public facilities, advocates for evidence-based practices would probably be well advised to meet often and frequently with public-sector mental health professionals and administrators. In this regard, it would probably also be judicious to include recovering persons in such discussions. Although we all should embrace maximization of choice and the rights of consumers to make mistakes, we also need to ensure that enthusiasm for the recovery model does not become so sweeping as to deny the benefits of scientific progress to persons who need treatment.

In summary, the main thesis of this article is that consumers who are more severely disabled, particularly in their decision making capacity, can best be treated with evidence-based approaches and perhaps with less attention to recovery-model considerations. However, for those whose mental illnesses become less disabling, the principles of the recovery model become increasingly applicable. ◆

References

1. The decade of the brain in its final year—and what a year it was! NAMI Advocate 21(4):1,3, May/June 2000

2. Torrey WC, Drake RE, Dixon L, et al: Implementing evidence-based practices for persons with severe mental illnesses. Psychiatric Services 52:45–50, 2001

3. Drake RE, Goldman HH, Leff HS, et al: Implementing evidence-based practices in routine mental health service settings. Psychiatric Services 52:179–182, 2001

4. Bond GR, Becker DR, Drake RE, et al: Implementing supported employment as an evidence-based practice. Psychiatric Services 52:313–322, 2001

5. Drake RE, Essock SM, Shaner A, et al: Implementing dual diagnosis services for clients with severe mental illness. Psychiatric Services 52:469–476, 2001

6. Minkoff K: Developing standards of care for individuals with co-occurring psychiatric and substance use disorders. Psychiatric Services 52:597–599, 2001

7. Mellman TA, Miller AL, Weissman EM, et al: Evidence-based pharmacologic treatment for people with severe mental illness: a focus on guidelines and algorithms. Psychiatric Services 52:619–625, 2001

8. Pelka F: Shrink resistant. Mainstream: Magazine of the Able-Disabled 22(9):22–27, 1998

9. Anthony W: Recovery from mental illness: the guiding vision of the mental health service system in the 1990s. Psychosocial Rehabilitation Journal 16(4):11–23, 1993

10. Sullivan P: Recovery from schizophrenia: what we can learn from the developing nations. Innovations and Research in Clinical Services, Community Support, and Rehabilitation 3(2):7–15, 1994

11. Beale V, Lambric T: The Recovery Concept: Implementation in the Mental Health System: A Report by the Community Support Program Advisory Committee. Columbus, Ohio, Ohio Department of Mental Health, Aug 1995:1–20

12. Jacobson N, Greenley D: What is recovery? A conceptual model and explication. Psychiatric Services 52:482–485, 2001

13. Peyser H: What is recovery? A commentary. Psychiatric Services 52:486–487, 2001

14. Munetz MR, Frese FJ: Getting ready for recovery: reconciling mandatory treatment with the recovery vision. Psychiatric Rehabilitation Journal 25(1):35–42, 2001

15. Szasz T: The Myth of Mental Illness. New York, Harper and Row, 1961

16. Deegan PE: Recovering our sense of value after being labeled mentally ill. Journal of Psychosocial Nursing 31(4):7–11, 1993

17. Deegan PE: The independent living movement and people with psychiatric disabilities: taking back control of our won lives. Psychosocial Rehabilitation Journal 15(3):3–19, 1992

18. Frese FJ: Cruising the cosmos: part three: psychosis and hospitalization: a consumer's recollection, in Surviving Mental Illness: Stress, Coping, and Adaptation. Edited by Hatfield AB, Lefley H. New York, Guilford, 1993

19. Frese FJ: A calling. Second Opinion 19(3): 11–25, 1994

20. Csernansky JG, Bardgett ME: Limbic-cortical neuronal damage and the pathophysiology of schizophrenia. Schizophrenia Bulletin 24:231–247, 1998

21. Frese FJ: Advocacy, recovery, and the challenges for consumerism for schizophrenia. Psychiatric Clinics of North America 21:233–249, 1998

22. Ross EC: NAMI campaign, policy team launch Omnibus Mental Illness Recovery Act. NAMI Advocate 20(4):1–5, 1999

23. Lehman AF, Steinwachs DM, survey coinvestigators of the PORT project: Translating research into practice: the Schizophrenia Patient Outcomes Research Team (PORT) treatment recommendations. Schizophrenia Bulletin 24:1–10, 1998

24. Pedon S: Learning From Our Past: Building Toward Our Future. Columbus, Ohio, NAMI Ohio, Dec 1999

25. North CS: Welcome Silence: My Triumph Over Schizophrenia. New York, Simon & Schuster, 1987

26. Fisher DB: Hope, humanity, and voice in recovery from psychiatric disability. Journal of the California Alliance for the Mentally Ill 5(3):7–11, 1994

27. Vogel-Scibilia S: Reflections on recovery. NAMI Advocate, winter:5,6, 2001

28. Bassman R: Consumers/survivors/ex-patients as change facilitators. New Directions for Mental Health Services, no 88:93–102, 2000

29. Siebert A: My transforming peak experience was diagnosed as schizophrenia. New Directions for Mental Health Services, no 88:103–111, 2000

30. Jamison KR: An Unquiet Mind: A Memoir of Moods and Madness. New York, Knopf, 1995

31. Frese FJ, Walker WW: The consumer-survivor movement, recovery, and consumer professionals. Professional Psychology: Research and Practice 28:243–245, 1997

32. Orrin D: How I earned my MSW despite my mental illness. Journal of the California Alliance for the Mentally Ill 8(2):61–63, 1997

33. Granger DA: Recovery from mental illness: a first person perspective of an emerging paradigm, in Recovery: The New Force in Mental Health. Columbus, Ohio, Ohio Department of Mental Health, Nov 1994

Implementing Supported Employment as an Evidence-Based Practice

Gary R. Bond, Ph.D.
Deborah R. Becker, M.Ed.
Robert E. Drake, M.D., Ph.D.
Charles A. Rapp, Ph.D.
Neil Meisler, M.S.W.
Anthony F. Lehman, M.D., M.S.P.H.
Morris D. Bell, Ph.D.
Crystal R. Blyler, Ph.D.

Supported employment for people with severe mental illness is an evidence-based practice, based on converging findings from eight randomized controlled trials and three quasi-experimental studies. The critical ingredients of supported employment have been well described, and a fidelity scale differentiates supported employment programs from other types of vocational services. The effectiveness of supported employment appears to be generalizable across a broad range of client characteristics and community settings. More research is needed on long-term outcomes and on cost-effectiveness. Access to supported employment programs remains a problem, despite their increasing use throughout the United States. The authors discuss barriers to implementation and strategies for overcoming them based on successful experiences in several states.

As a result of more than two decades of research, we know a great deal about improving outcomes and enhancing the recovery process for persons with severe mental illness by providing effective mental health services. Unfortunately, the implementation of interventions that have been shown to be effective by research, termed here evidence-based practices, lags considerably behind the state of knowledge. Individuals with severe mental disorders such as schizophrenia are unlikely to receive treatment with basic evidence-based practices in routine mental health settings (1). Implementation of evidence-based practices must overcome many obstacles, some generic and some specific to a particular evidence-based practice. Nevertheless, the field of mental health services is slowly committing itself to providing research-based services as the foundation of care (2).

In this paper, the first of several on specific evidence-based practices for persons with severe mental illness, we discuss supported employment, a recent approach to vocational rehabilitation that has proved to be consistently more effective than traditional approaches. Our goals are to familiarize clients, families, clinicians, administrators, and mental health policy makers with supported employment; to review the findings and limitations of current research; and to discuss implementation issues, including availability, barriers, and strategies. Because several recent reviews of research on supported employment already exist (3–7), our intent is to provide information that is accessible to stakeholder groups other than researchers.

Supported employment

Supported employment is a well-defined approach to helping people with disabilities participate as much as possible in the competitive labor market, working in jobs they prefer with the level of professional help they need. According to the federal definition, supported employment means "competitive work in integrated work settings . . . consistent with the strengths, resources, priorities, concerns, abilities, capabilities, interests, and informed choice of the individuals, for individuals with the most significant disabilities for whom competitive employment has not traditionally occurred; or for whom competitive employment has been interrupted or intermittent as a result of a significant disability" (8).

Although the federal definition of supported employment includes ref-

Dr. Bond is affiliated with the department of psychology at Indiana University–Purdue University Indianapolis, 402 North Blackford Street, Indianapolis, Indiana 46202 (e-mail, gbond@iupui.edu). Ms. Becker and Dr. Drake are with the New Hampshire–Dartmouth Psychiatric Research Center in Lebanon, New Hampshire. Dr. Rapp is affiliated with the School of Social Welfare at the University of Kansas in Lawrence. Mr. Meisler is with the department of psychiatry at the Medical University of South Carolina in Charleston. Dr. Lehman is with the department of psychiatry at the University of Maryland in Baltimore. Dr. Bell is with the department of psychiatry at Yale University in New Haven, Connecticut. Dr. Blyler is affiliated with the Center for Mental Health Services of the Substance Abuse and Mental Health Services Administration in Rockville, Maryland. This article was originally published in the March 2001 issue of Psychiatric Services.

erence to transitional employment, that is, temporary community job placements, the two are very different, both conceptually and in practice (9). Many agencies offer both, and when they do, practitioners understand them to be different approaches; transitional employment is seen as a step toward supported employment (10). We do not discuss transitional employment in this paper.

Although many supported employment principles have been espoused for decades (11), these ideas crystallized in the 1980s through the efforts of a national network of educators, who concluded that sheltered workshops isolate people with developmental disabilities from mainstream society (12). This network was successful in changing federal regulations on the types of services funded by the federal-state vocational rehabilitation system.

By 1987 supported employment had attracted attention in the psychiatric rehabilitation field (13). As adapted for this population, supported employment programs typically provide individual placements in competitive employment—that is, community jobs paying at least minimum wage that any person can apply for—in accord with client choices and capabilities, without requiring extended prevocational training. Unlike other vocational approaches (4,14), supported employment programs do not screen people for work readiness, but help all who say they want to work; they do not provide intermediate work experiences, such as prevocational work units, transitional employment, or sheltered workshops; they actively facilitate job acquisition, often sending staff to accompany clients on interviews; and they provide ongoing support once the client is employed.

Supported employment programs are found in a wide variety of service contexts, including community mental health centers, community rehabilitation programs, clubhouses, and psychiatric rehabilitation centers (10, 15,16). Although the evidence suggests that supported employment is optimally effective only when clients concurrently receive adequate case management, it is not necessarily lim-

ited to a specific service model such as assertive community treatment.

The most comprehensively described supported employment approach for people with severe mental illness is the individual placement and support model (17,18). We do not view this approach as a distinct supported employment model. Instead, it is intended as a standardization of supported employment principles in programs for people with severe mental illness, so that supported employment can be clearly described, scientifically studied, and implemented in communities. In fact, a survey of 116 supported employment programs throughout the United States found that these programs generally follow principles of the individual placement and support model (19).

Effectiveness of supported employment

To understand the context of the current review, several points from the broader vocational literature are critical. First, interventions that do not target job placement directly have very little impact on employment outcomes (20). Second, many vocational approaches to helping people with severe mental illness gain employment have been developed over the past half century. Few have been evaluated rigorously; those that have been examined in controlled trials have yielded disappointing results (4,14,21,22).

Quasi-experimental studies. To date, three quasi-experimental studies have evaluated day treatment programs that converted their rehabilitation services to supported employment. Drake and colleagues (23) studied a rural New Hampshire community mental health center that developed a supported employment program to replace the day treatment services. A natural experiment compared the conversion site with a nearby site, which continued its day treatment along with traditional brokered vocational services. The competitive employment rate increased substantially at the conversion site, whereas the rate was unchanged at the comparison site. Moreover, adverse outcomes such as hospitalization, incarceration, and dropouts did not increase at the conversion site.

Clients, their families, and mental health staff had favorable reactions to the conversion, although a minority mentioned loss of social contact as a drawback (24). Interestingly, many clients who did not find work also reported that they benefited from the change because they discovered satisfying activities outside the community mental health center.

Replacing day treatment with supported employment also led to cost savings (25). Given the success of the initial conversion, the second site subsequently converted to supported employment with similarly favorable results (26). In a second study involving the downsizing of a day treatment program in a small city, clients who transferred to a new supported employment program had better outcomes than those who remained in day treatment (27).

A third study compared two Rhode Island day treatment programs that converted to supported employment with one that did not (28), with similar findings. Others have also reported successful conversions of day treatment to supported employment programs (29). These evaluations demonstrate that supported employment can be implemented in a cost-effective manner in real-world settings with a broad range of clients with severe mental illness, not just a select group who sign up for supported employment.

Randomized controlled trials. A 1997 review (3) summarized the findings of six randomized controlled trials comparing supported employment with a variety of traditional vocational services for people with severe mental illness (30–35). All six studies reported significant gains in obtaining and keeping employment for persons enrolled in supported employment. For example, a mean of 58 percent of supported employment clients achieved competitive employment at some time over a 12- to 18-month period, compared with 21 percent of the control group, who received a range of alternative vocational interventions, including skills training, sheltered work, and vocational counseling as steps toward competitive job placement. Control subjects received what providers in their communities believed to be best practices in vocational rehabilitation.

Other competitive employment outcomes, such as time employed and employment earnings, also favored supported employment clients over those in control groups. A meta-analysis of these studies reached very similar conclusions, noting that the findings were robust (5,6).

Recently, data collection was completed for the Center for Mental Health Services Employment Intervention Demonstration Program (36). Eight sites in this project used randomized controlled trials to evaluate the effectiveness of supported employment. Reports of findings from this multicenter trial are expected over the next year.

Two sites have reported preliminary experimental findings. In Hartford, Connecticut, Mueser and associates (37) compared individual placement and support with two established vocational approaches. One was a psychiatric rehabilitation center using transitional employment, and the other was a brokered approach using a combination of sheltered workshops, government set-aside jobs, and individual placements. Meisler and colleagues (38) compared an individual placement and support program working within an assertive community treatment team with usual vocational services in a rural community in South Carolina. The control group was assigned to a well-respected rehabilitation center with long-term contracts providing numerous government set-aside jobs.

Findings from both studies replicated the previous findings of large differences in competitive employment outcomes favoring supported employment over traditional approaches. Even with protected jobs—transitional employment and set-aside jobs—factored in, supported employment clients in both studies still had better employment outcomes.

Many of these studies have also examined nonvocational outcomes, such as rehospitalization rates, symptoms, quality of life, and self-esteem. Studies rarely have found any experimental differences in nonvocational outcomes favoring clients enrolled in

supported employment programs over those in comparison programs. In other words, the group effects for supported employment programs appear to be restricted mainly to competitive employment outcomes, at least for the relatively brief follow-up periods in the studies reviewed. However, neither has any research suggested any adverse effects from participation in supported employment programs. Rehospitalization rates are unaffected by participation in supported employment, contrary to the belief that the stress of work might lead to higher relapse rates.

Although enrollment in a supported employment program itself does not lead to improved nonvocational outcomes, clients who actually engage in competitive work do experience improvements in self-esteem and in control of symptoms, compared with clients who do not work or work minimally (39,40).

Cost considerations are a core issue in decisions to implement psychiatric services. Supported employment services are labor intensive. Annual cost per supported employment participant is around $2,000 to $4,000 (25,41). These figures are similar to those for traditional vocational services (42). Clients enrolled in supported employment programs sometimes use fewer mental health services, notably day treatment, suggesting a cost offset (25,43–45).

Critical components

Reviewers seeking to identify empirically validated principles of supported employment have reached similar conclusions (7,46–49). Certain components are almost always present in successful vocational programs. They are generally found in the supported employment programs evaluated in the eight randomized controlled trials summarized above. The following components are predictive of better employment outcomes:

♦ The agency providing supported employment services is committed to competitive employment as an attainable goal for its clients with severe mental illness, devoting its resources for rehabilitation services to this endeavor rather than to day treatment or sheltered work. Numerous studies

indicate that this element is common in successful programs (23,26–29,33, 31,10,50).

♦ Supported employment programs use a rapid job search approach to help clients obtain jobs directly, rather than providing lengthy preemployment assessment, training, and counseling. The evidence in this area is strong, with two randomized controlled trials focusing specifically on this variable (30,51), plus five randomized controlled trials in which this component was a critical difference between study conditions (32–34,37,38). A randomized controlled trial evaluating a vocational approach involving extended classroom training before job placement yielded employment outcomes similar to those of a control group referred to the state vocational rehabilitation office for vocational services (52).

♦ Staff and clients find individualized job placements according to client preferences, strengths, and work experiences. Several correlational studies support this conclusion (49,53–56).

♦ Follow-along supports are maintained indefinitely. Correlational findings from four different research groups indicate that this component is an important one (31,57–59).

♦ The supported employment program is closely integrated with the mental health treatment team. The experimental evidence is consistent with this conclusion even though this variable has not been studied in isolation (31–33,35,37,38,59). This principle is also supported by a strong theoretical rationale (60). However, despite its strong evidence base, it is not universally practiced (19).

Together these principles serve as a foundation for evidence-based guidelines for providing effective supported employment services. In one statewide survey, programs rated high in implementing these principles had better employment outcomes (unpublished data, Becker DR, 2000). A number of specific program elements—for example, reasonable caseload size, diverse employment settings, assertive outreach, and benefits counseling—are found in most supported employment programs (15), but the association between these elements and better employment outcomes has not yet been established. Further research is needed to clarify the critical ingredients of supported employment, which will lead to modifications, refinements, and additions.

Limitations of the evidence
Client factors
The most consistent finding from the supported employment literature has been the absence of specific client factors predicting better employment outcomes. Diagnosis, symptoms, age, gender, disability status, prior hospitalization, and education have been examined, and none have proved to be strong or consistent predictors (30,32,33). Notably, a co-occurring condition of substance use has not been found to predict employment outcomes (61–63).

Although a work history predicts better employment outcomes in supported employment programs, supported employment remains more effective than traditional vocational services for clients with both good and poor work histories (28,32,33). We speculate that the professional assistance provided by supported employment programs at every stage of the employment process compensates for client deficits in a way that less assertive vocational rehabilitation approaches do not. Consequently, the extensive literature on client predictors of work outcomes among people with severe mental illness who either have had little vocational assistance or have been enrolled in traditional vocational programs (48) may be largely irrelevant for supported employment programs.

Randomized controlled trials of supported employment have been conducted in settings with significant numbers of Caucasian (30–32,59), African-American (33,38), and Latino (37) clients. Although more replications are needed, all the evidence to date suggests that the greater effectiveness of supported employment compared with traditional vocational services is generalizable to both the African-American and Latino populations. Within-study comparisons of employment rates for different ethnic groups have been hampered by small sample sizes, so we cannot yet determine whether supported employment is equally effective for all ethnic groups within a specific setting.

We may make our best progress in understanding the role of ethnicity in supported employment programs by combining results across studies using meta-analytic techniques and through qualitative studies (64–66). We know anecdotally that culture and language pose significant barriers to providing supported employment in some populations.

Not all clients benefit from supported employment. For example, in community mental health centers converting day treatment programs to supported employment programs, some clients do not have employment as a current goal; not surprisingly, these clients usually do not work. But even among clients who express an interest in working, a sizable proportion are not working at any given time. We need to develop effective strategies for these clients. Helping clients decide whether supported employment is right for them also is critical. Informational sessions explaining beforehand how supported employment works improve clients' ability to make informed decisions about participating, thereby potentially reducing dropout rates (67,68).

Community and economic factors
Supported employment has been implemented successfully in many different types of communities. Programs in rural areas are no less successful than those in urban areas (49,50). One counterintuitive finding is that economic conditions apparently do not have a potent influence on employment rates for a supported employment program (50,69–71). Catalano and colleagues (69) have speculated that an economic theory of labor markets applies here. The primary labor market, comprising professional and semiprofessional jobs, shrinks during economic recessions. The secondary labor market, which includes entry-level jobs in the service industry, is more elastic and less vulnerable to economic downturns. Supported employment programs find jobs mostly in this secondary labor market, where jobs are usually available.

However, the aforementioned studies examined a relatively restricted range of unemployment. The findings may not be generalizable to communities where the unemployment rate is very high (35).

Job opportunities available to clients with severe mental illness are often restricted because of the clients' limited work experience, education, and training, and consequently most supported employment jobs are unskilled (3,72). Half of all clients leave their supported employment positions within six months (3), although nondisabled workers in these occupations also have high turnover rates (73). Moreover, most supported employment positions are part-time. Clients often limit work hours to avoid jeopardizing Social Security and Medicaid benefits (48,74). A continuing challenge for supported employment programs is helping clients capitalize on educational and training opportunities so that they may qualify for skilled jobs and develop satisfying careers (72).

Program factors
Specific details about the best ways to provide supported employment services have not been adequately researched. Issues include the role of disclosure of mental illness in finding and keeping jobs, the range, location, timing, and intensity of supports provided to clients (57,75), and the nature of coworker and supervisor supports (76). The relationship between supported employment services and medication issues has not been well studied despite its assumed importance (77).

Long-term outcomes of supported employment also have not been widely studied. Programs that remain engaged with their clients over time, respond to clients' expressed wishes, and sustain an approach that integrates clinical and rehabilitation services are those we believe have the best outcomes over time. However, with few exceptions (30,58,59), most randomized controlled trials do not have follow-up information beyond two years. Much longer follow-up periods are needed to determine whether sustained commitment can yield favorable outcomes for more clients.

Implementation barriers

Access to supported employment

Sixty to 70 percent of people with severe mental illness would like to work in competitive employment (78,79), yet 85 percent or more of those in public mental health systems are not doing so (78–82). Most prefer competitive employment to sheltered workshops (83) and day treatment (30,84). However, most clients lack access to employment services of any kind. Less than 25 percent of clients with severe mental illness receive any form of vocational assistance (1,85, 86), and only a fraction of these clients have access to supported employment (87). In some states, supported employment programs are now commonly found in community mental health centers, but their capacity falls far short of the need (19, 50). A further question concerns the quality of available programs. Not surprisingly, it is mixed (15,49).

Barriers to implementation of high-quality programs exist at many levels—within federal, state, and local governments and program or clinic administrations, among clinicians and supervisors, and in the collaboration with clients or families. The remainder of this paper is devoted to discussing the barriers to implementing high-quality supported employment programs and offering suggestions based on experience for overcoming them.

Government barriers

Historically, the federal-state vocational rehabilitation system has been the primary funding source for employment services. However, federal funding for vocational rehabilitation has never been sufficient to serve more than a tiny proportion of the population in need (88). Moreover, many observers have expressed doubts about whether this funding has been used wisely. Vocational rehabilitation expenditures apparently have been disproportionately devoted to administration and to assessment and other preemployment activities (89). Compounding the problem is the fact that persons with severe mental illness fail to complete the vocational rehabilitation eligibility process twice as often as people with

physical disabilities (90). Nevertheless, vocational rehabilitation agencies continue to allocate minimal funding for supported employment services (91).

Public funding for mental health is a second source for financing supported employment services. Unfortunately, community mental health centers historically have allocated only a tiny proportion of their budgets to vocational services (85). Since the 1980s, most states have amended their Medicaid state plans to cover community mental health services under the optional rehabilitative services provision, which permits a broad interpretation of the range of reimbursable interventions.

Vocational training is among the few services statutorily excluded from Medicaid reimbursement. However, evidence-based components of supported employment, such as ongoing supportive counseling in home and community-based settings, team meetings, psychiatrist involvement in rehabilitation planning, and assisting clients in developing job opportunities, are all Medicaid-reimbursed rehabilitative services that states may cover. Yet most state Medicaid plans include unnecessary limitations on covered services when they involve vocational activities. Given the increasing proportion of total funding of community mental health services that Medicaid expenditures represent, misinterpretation of federal Medicaid policy results in a major barrier to supported employment service access.

Fee-for-service systems of reimbursement for units of service, regardless of outcomes, have created incentives to perpetuate services that are not evidence based, such as day treatment (92). Some commentators have concluded that financing of supported employment programs within managed care systems will not be any easier (93).

The fragmentation of supported employment funding has also resulted in separation of services. Historically, supported employment services have been brokered—that is, offered at an agency separate from the community mental health center (16)—even though we now know that this

approach is counterproductive (47, 60). Even supported employment programs that are located in community mental health centers often are not closely integrated with mental health treatment teams (19), despite strong evidence that such integration is vital for success. In Indiana, a separate role for follow-along specialists created by separate funding sources has contributed to discontinuity of services (94).

Directors of state mental health departments can have a critical leadership role in promoting supported employment services. In the 1980s, Ohio's decision to pursue case management and housing as top priorities led to critical improvements, but this decision sacrificed the development of employment services by relegating it to a secondary goal (82). Some states have adopted a "range of vocational options" (95), leading to a proliferation of diverse—and untested—models, whereas other states have invested major resources in specific models that are not evidence based. Still other states have taken the stance that supported employment is not the business of the state mental health agency. Moreover, most states do not systematically monitor client outcomes, precluding the development of objective methods for rewarding successful employment programs.

Program administrators

From an administrator's perspective, common barriers include finding money to finance start-up and ongoing program costs, managing organizational change, and coping with political ramifications of change in the community. Administrators often do not provide the leadership for the adoption of innovations, even when they are evidence based. Administrators who do not have information about evidence-based practices may not value their outcomes or believe that they are possible (49). Administrators, especially those who received training and professional experience in an earlier era, may hold negativist attitudes about the feasibility of work—for example, "Schizophrenia is a chronic disease with little hope of recovery . . . work is a source of unnecessary stress."

If administrators are unwilling to consider change, it is unlikely that practitioners will. Poor management practices constitute another obvious barrier to implementation of evidence-based practices (96). Agencies that are driven by crises and chaos often have leaders and supervisors who have not established a system of careful treatment planning that is related to clients' desires and needs.

Clinicians and supervisors

Like administrators, clinicians often view clients as too unmotivated to work (97) and often underestimate the need for vocational services (98,99). Many practitioners lack adequate information and skills to staff supported employment programs (100–102).

Resistance to change is a barrier in any organization. In the mental health field, professional identities are defined by what practitioners do—methods employed, program name, and the like—or by their discipline, not by the outcomes sought. Program changes sometimes are introduced as externally imposed ideas rather than resulting from a process that includes the participation of the clinicians and supervisors, who are ultimately responsible for implementing the desired change (103). In such circumstances, practitioners perceive change efforts as a criticism and devaluing of their work.

Another common barrier concerns inadequate resources. Staff members cannot implement supported employment programs effectively if they do not have enough time to carry out their duties or if supervisors give them conflicting messages about the scope of their responsibilities. For example, when employment specialists are assigned additional job duties that are not vocational, they are distracted from the employment effort.

Clients and families

Clients and family members often do not have accurate information about supported employment. Sometimes clients are discouraged from considering employment by well-meaning clinicians and family members who believe that the stress associated with work outweighs the benefits. Instead, they are directed to day programs.

Clients often believe that returning to work automatically compromises their eligibility for Social Security and Medicaid benefits. Families may not be given information on how to support a family member's work efforts, or they may not be considered part of the team or support network.

Strategies for implementation

Although we have more systematic information about barriers to evidence-based practices than we do about strategies to overcome them, some approaches for implementing evidence-based practices have been identified (104,105).

Government efforts

At the state level, a first step is to set clear outcome priorities. Next, systematic assessment of employment outcomes is absolutely essential. State mental health authorities must remove organizational and financial barriers to the development of supported employment programs, as has been done in New Hampshire (50), Vermont (unpublished data, Dalmasse D, 1998), Rhode Island (106), and Kansas (49). In both New Hampshire and Rhode Island, state mental health and Medicaid agencies joined to request that the Health Care Financing Administration allow reimbursement for supported employment services aside from direct interventions to teach job skills. Their requests were approved, thereby enabling Medicaid financing to greatly increase clients' access to supported employment services.

Recent federal legislation—the Medicaid buy-in program authorized by the Balanced Budget Act of 1997 and the Ticket to Work and Work Incentives Improvement Act of 1999—has permitted state governments more flexibility in establishing Medicaid eligibility, with the intent of reducing barriers to employment posed by the potential loss of Medicaid benefits (107). Some states—Oregon and Minnesota, for example—have implemented new policies expanding Medicaid coverage to allow more liberal income and resource thresholds for people with disabilities who work.

State mental health authorities have had success in providing direct incen-

tives to local systems for meeting employment goals. In Ohio, participating systems doubled their employment rate when incentives were instituted (82). In New Hampshire, the competitive employment rate for community mental health center clients with severe mental illness has increased from 7 percent to 37 percent since 1990, when the state began emphasizing competitive employment in contracting (50). State vocational rehabilitation agencies in Alabama, Oklahoma, and Pennsylvania have initiated "results-based funding" for supported employment, which similarly rewards agencies for performance (108,109). Some caution is necessary, because unless designed carefully, such incentive systems may encourage enrolling clients with the fewest needs.

Incentives are not enough, however. The state agencies should also take the leadership in providing technical assistance by forming partnerships with leading research and training centers with appropriate expertise, as have those of New Hampshire (110), Rhode Island (106), and other states. Kansas, Indiana, New Jersey, and New York City have established supported employment technical assistance centers to help local programs implement and monitor supported employment services.

Building consensus among stakeholders is another element in the adoption of evidence-based practices. The National Association of State Mental Health Program Directors has issued a position statement on employment and rehabilitation for persons with severe psychiatric disabilities that identifies state mental health agencies as having a responsibility to influence vocational rehabilitation and other state employment agencies to collaborate to improve access by persons with severe mental illness to competitive employment (111). Accepting this mandate, Rhode Island's state mental health agency has involved the state's Medicaid and vocational rehabilitation agencies in funding supported employment. Funding for consensus-building activities related to exemplary practices is available through the Community Action Grant Program of the Center for Mental Health Services.

Efforts of program administrators

High-achieving organizations concentrate energy and resources on specific outcomes and reduce distractions to those outcomes (112). Important elements of leadership include articulating desired outcomes and practices for achieving them, building an organizational structure and culture that will facilitate implementing evidence-based practices, designing systems to monitor evidence-based practices and client outcomes, hiring staff with appropriate attitudes and skills, establishing group supervision or other methods of collaboration, creating employee evaluation procedures that emphasize evidence-based practices and employment outcomes, and providing rewards for high performance in those areas (49,113).

Supported employment programs are most successful in agencies that make a total commitment to competitive employment without diluting their focus and resources with traditional forms of vocational programming (49,50). A similar pattern is found in the developmental disability field, where supported employment has failed to develop its full potential because many agencies have viewed supported employment as an "add-on" service while maintaining large sheltered workshops (114).

As noted above, community mental health centers have been successful in converting day treatment programs completely to supported employment. Because this redeployment of resources has the advantage of cost savings in addition to acceptance by important stakeholders, it is a very appealing strategy. Consumer-run services can play a role in meeting the social needs of unemployed clients after conversion from day treatment to supported employment (115).

Monitoring the fidelity of program implementation is critical for implementing evidence-based practices (116). Accordingly, researchers, state planners, program directors, clients, and family members are increasingly emphasizing fidelity. The Individual Placement and Support Fidelity Scale (117), a 15-item instrument that assesses the implementation of critical ingredients of supported employment, is one such tool in the public

domain. Although it was designed for use by assessors who are familiar with the critical ingredients of the model, its simplicity permits its use by nonresearchers.

Adequate reliability has been found in a field test using site visits by pairs of assessors who interviewed staff, studied charts, and observed program activities (117). The Individual Placement and Support Fidelity Scale clearly differentiates supported employment programs from other vocational approaches, suggesting that it can be used to determine whether a program actually is implementing supported employment (19). More comprehensive scales measuring supported employment implementation also have been field-tested (15,94).

Efforts of clinicians and supervisors

Agencies that successfully adopt supported employment appear to share a set of common elements (49,113, 118). Successful programs give staff the resources they need to do their job well. This also means that the agency itself must be well managed in other areas and must provide high-quality case management services. Supervisors need to provide clear vision, organize services into a multidisciplinary team structure, and focus on outcomes rather than service units and paperwork (119).

Community mental health centers successfully adopting an innovation usually have at least one key change agent who champions the innovation (120). The change agent must have sufficient authority to implement change. When introducing supported employment, the change agent identifies respected frontline practitioners who can help lead the implementation effort. They in turn recruit other staff to join in the planning and development of the new program so that all staff will feel ownership of the program.

Adequate training and ongoing supervision are critical to give staff the skills to implement the practice (118). Guidelines, training manuals, and videotapes are important tools for ongoing monitoring and transmission of the culture of the supported employment program (118). Another critical element is expert consultation

through site visits and telephone conference calls. Implementation is facilitated by having staff—not just employment specialists but also administrators, clinicians, and supervisors—visit exemplary supported employment programs.

Efforts of clients and families

Clients and families are well aware of the need for vocational services (89,98,121) but need to know what good services look like and how to advocate effectively in legislation and funding decisions. They can have influence over setting standards and ensuring adherence to those standards at the state, program, and client levels. Clients and family members should seek membership on advisory boards at all levels. They can collaborate with state officials to fund supported employment programs and to establish standards based on evidence-based practices and have them incorporated in licensing standards, requests for proposals for grant funds, and so on. At the program level, they can demand that entrance criteria for supported employment be based on a client's desire to work and not on symptoms or work history. They can also participate in designing supported employment programs. On an individual client level, they can argue for client choice and services that match evidence-based practices.

Conclusions

The emerging evidence base on supported employment is clear and consistent, with improved employment outcomes across many different types of settings and populations. In addition, most supported employment approaches described in the literature converge on a set of critical components.

One key remaining task is to overcome implementation barriers to make supported employment services available on a widespread basis. No other vocational rehabilitation approach for people with severe mental illness has attained the status of evidence-based practice despite a half century of program innovation and informal experimentation by many psychiatric rehabilitation programs. Proponents of other vocational approaches either have failed to empirically investigate their methods or have failed to find strong evidence. It is also true that many vocational program approaches that are not effective continue to be widely practiced.

Beyond implementing supported employment, we must continue to refine and improve our model to reach a wider spectrum of the population and to help clients not only find and keep paid community jobs but also to develop long-term careers. ♦

Acknowledgments

Work on this paper was supported by National Institute of Mental Health grants MH-00842 and MH-00839, Center for Mental Health Services contract 280-00-8049, and a grant from the Robert Wood Johnson Foundation.

References

1. Lehman AF, Steinwachs DM: Patterns of usual care for schizophrenia: initial results from the Schizophrenia Patient Outcomes Research Team (PORT) client survey. Schizophrenia Bulletin 24:11–23, 1998

2. Drake RE, Goldman HH, Leff HS, et al: Implementing evidence-based practices in routine mental health service settings. Psychiatric Services 52:179–182, 2001

3. Bond GR, Drake RE, Mueser KT, et al: An update on supported employment for people with severe mental illness. Psychiatric Services 48:335–346, 1997

4. Bond GR, Drake RE, Becker DR, et al: Effectiveness of psychiatric rehabilitation approaches for employment of people with severe mental illness. Journal of Disability Policy Studies 10(1):18–52, 1999

5. Crowther R, Marshall M, Bond GR, et al: Vocational rehabilitation for people with severe mental disorders. Cochrane Review, in Cochrane Library. Oxford, England, Update Software, in press

6. Crowther RE, Marshall M, Bond GR, et al: Helping people with severe mental illness to return to work: a systematic review. British Medical Journal, in press

7. Ridgway P, Rapp C: The Active Ingredients in Achieving Competitive Employment for People With Psychiatric Disabilities: A Research Synthesis. Lawrence, University of Kansas, School of Social Welfare, 1998

8. Rehabilitation Act Amendments of 1998: Title IV of the Workforce Investment Act of 1998, Pub Law 105-220, 112 Stat 936

9. Bilby R: A response to the criticisms of transitional employment. Psychosocial Rehabilitation Journal 16(2):69–82, 1992

10. Picone J, Drake RE, Becker D, et al: A survey of clubhouse programs. Indianapolis, Indiana University Purdue University Indianapolis, Department of Psychology, 1998

11. Newman L: Instant placement: a new model for providing rehabilitation services within a community mental health program. Community Mental Health Journal 6:401–410, 1970

12. Wehman P: Supported competitive employment for persons with severe disabilities. Journal of Applied Rehabilitation Counseling 17:24–29, 1986

13. Mellen V, Danley K: Special issue: Supported Employment for Persons with Severe Mental Illness. Psychosocial Rehabilitation Journal 9(2):1–102, 1987

14. Bond GR: Vocational rehabilitation, in Handbook of Psychiatric Rehabilitation. Edited by Liberman RP. New York, Macmillan, 1992

15. Bond GR, Picone J, Mauer B, et al: The Quality of Supported Employment Implementation Scale. Journal of Vocational Rehabilitation 14:201–212, 2000

16. Gervey R, Parrish A, Bond GR: Survey of exemplary supported employment programs for persons with psychiatric disabilities. Journal of Vocational Rehabilitation 5:115–125, 1995

17. Becker DR, Drake RE: A Working Life: The Individual Placement and Support (IPS) Program. Concord, NH, New Hampshire–Dartmouth Psychiatric Research Center, 1993

18. Drake RE, Becker DR: The individual placement and support model of supported employment. Psychiatric Services 47:473–475, 1996

19. Bond GR, Vogler KM, Resnick SG, et al: Dimensions of supported employment: factor structure of the IPS Fidelity Scale. Journal of Mental Health, in press

20. Vandergoot D: Review of placement research literature: implications for research and practice. Rehabilitation Counseling Bulletin 30:243–272, 1987

21. Baronet A, Gerber GJ: Psychiatric rehabilitation: efficacy of four models. Clinical Psychology Review 18:189–228, 1998

22. Lehman AF: Vocational rehabilitation in schizophrenia. Schizophrenia Bulletin 21:645–656, 1995

23. Drake RE, Becker DR, Biesanz JC, et al: Rehabilitation day treatment vs supported employment: I. vocational outcomes. Community Mental Health Journal 30:519–532, 1994

24. Torrey WC, Becker DR, Drake RE: Rehabilitative day treatment versus supported employment: II. consumer, family, and staff reactions to a program change. Psychosocial Rehabilitation Journal 18(3):67–75, 1995

25. Clark RE: Supported employment and managed care: can they co-exist? Psychiatric Rehabilitation Journal 22(1):62–68, 1998

26. Drake RE, Becker DR, Biesanz JC, et al: Day treatment versus supported employment for persons with severe mental illness: a replication study. Psychiatric Services 47:1125–1127, 1996

27. Bailey EL, Ricketts SK, Becker DR, et al: Do long-term day treatment clients benefit from supported employment? Psychiatric Rehabilitation Journal 22(1):24–29, 1998

28. Becker DR, Bond GR, McCarthy D, et al: Converting day treatment centers to supported employment programs in Rhode Island. Psychiatric Services 52:351–357, 2001

29. Gold M, Marrone J: Mass Bay Employment Services (a service of Bay Cove Human Services, Inc): a story of leadership, vision, and action resulting in employment for people with mental illness, in Roses and Thorns from the Grassroots. Boston, Institute of Community Action, 1998

30. Bond GR, Dietzen LL, McGrew JH, et al: Accelerating entry into supported employment for persons with severe psychiatric disabilities. Rehabilitation Psychology 40:91–111, 1995

31. Chandler D, Meisel J, Hu T, et al: A capitated model for a cross-section of severely mentally ill clients: employment outcomes. Community Mental Health Journal 33:501–516, 1997

32. Drake RE, McHugo GJ, Becker DR, et al: The New Hampshire study of supported employment for people with severe mental illness: vocational outcomes. Journal of Consulting and Clinical Psychology 64:391–399, 1996

33. Drake RE, McHugo GJ, Bebout RR, et al: A randomized clinical trial of supported employment for inner-city patients with severe mental illness. Archives of General Psychiatry 56:627–633, 1999

34. Gervey R, Bedell JR: Supported employment in vocational rehabilitation, in Psychological Assessment and Treatment of Persons With Severe Mental Disorders. Edited by Bedell JR. Washington, DC, Taylor & Francis, 1994

35. McFarlane WR, Dushay RA, Deakins SM, et al: Employment outcomes in family-aided assertive community treatment. American Journal of Orthopsychiatry 70:203–214, 2000

36. Carey MA: The continuing need for research on vocational rehabilitation programs. Psychosocial Rehabilitation Journal 18(4):163–164, 1995

37. Mueser KT, Clark RE, Drake RE, et al: A comparison of the individual placement and support model with the psychosocial rehabilitation approach to vocational rehabilitation for consumers with severe mental illness: the results of a controlled trial. Presented at the Fourth Biennial Research Seminar on Work, Matrix Research Institute, Philadelphia, Oct 11–13, 2000

38. Meisler N, Williams O, Kelleher J, et al: Rural-based supported employment approaches: results from South Carolina site of the Employment Intervention Demonstration Project. Presented at the Fourth Biennial Research Seminar on Work, Matrix Research Institute, Philadelphia, Oct 11–13, 2000

39. Bond GR, Resnick SR, Drake RE, et al: Does competitive employment improve nonvocational outcomes for people with severe mental illness? Journal of Consulting

and Clinical Psychology, in press

40. Mueser KT, Becker DR, Torrey WC, et al: Work and nonvocational domains of functioning in persons with severe mental illness: a longitudinal analysis. Journal of Nervous and Mental Disease 185:419–426, 1997

41. Kregel J, Wehman P, Revell G, et al: Supported employment benefit-cost analysis: preliminary findings. Journal of Vocational Rehabilitation 14:153–161, 2000

42. Clark RE, Bond GR: Costs and benefits of vocational programs for people with serious mental illness, in Schizophrenia. Edited by Moscarelli M, Rupp A, Sartorius N. Sussex, England, Wiley, 1996

43. Bond GR, Dietzen LL, Vogler KM, et al: Toward a framework for evaluating costs and benefits of psychiatric rehabilitation: three case examples. Journal of Vocational Rehabilitation 5:75–88, 1995

44. Clark RE, Xie H, Becker DR, et al: Benefits and costs of supported employment from three perspectives. Journal of Behavioral Health Services and Research 25:22–34, 1998

45. Rogers ES, Sciarappa K, MacDonald-Wilson K, et al: A benefit-cost analysis of a supported employment model for persons with psychiatric disabilities. Evaluation and Program Planning 18:105–115, 1995

46. Bond GR: Applying psychiatric rehabilitation principles to employment: recent findings, in Schizophrenia: Exploring the Spectrum of Psychosis. Edited by Ancill RJ, Holliday S, Higenbottam J. Chichester, England, Wiley, 1994

47. Bond GR: Principles of the individual placement and support model: empirical support. Psychiatric Rehabilitation Journal 22(1):11–23, 1998

48. Cook J, Razzano L: Vocational rehabilitation for persons with schizophrenia: recent research and implications for practice. Schizophrenia Bulletin 26:87–103, 2000

49. Gowdy EA: "Work Is the Best Medicine I Can Have": Identifying Best Practices in Supported Employment for People With Psychiatric Disabilities. Ph.D. dissertation. Lawrence, University of Kansas, School of Social Welfare, 2000

50. Drake RE, Fox TS, Leather PK, et al: Regional variation in competitive employment for persons with severe mental illness. Administration and Policy in Mental Health 25:493–504, 1998

51. Bond GR, Dincin J: Accelerating entry into transitional employment in a psychosocial rehabilitation agency. Rehabilitation Psychology 31:143–155, 1986

52. Rogers ES: A randomized controlled study of psychiatric vocational rehabilitation services. Presented at the Fourth Biennial Research Seminar on Work, Matrix Research Institute, Philadelphia, Oct 11–13, 2000

53. Abrams K, DonAroma P, Karan OC: Consumer choice as a predictor of job satisfaction and supervisor ratings for people with disabilities. Journal of Vocational Rehabilitation 9:205–215, 1997

54. Becker DR, Drake RE, Farabaugh A, et al: Job preferences of clients with severe psychiatric disorders participating in supported employment programs. Psychiatric Services 47:1223–1226, 1996

55. Gervey R, Kowal H: A description of a model for placing youth and young adults with psychiatric disabilities in competitive employment. Presented at the International Association of Psychosocial Rehabilitation Services Conference, Albuquerque, May 9–13, 1994

56. Mueser KT, Becker DR, Wolfe R: Supported employment, job preferences, and job tenure and satisfaction. Journal of Mental Health, in press

57. Cook JA, Razzano L: Natural vocational supports for persons with severe mental illness: thresholds supported competitive employment program. New Directions for Mental Health Services, no 56:23–41, 1992

58. McHugo GJ, Drake RE, Becker DR: The durability of supported employment effects. Psychiatric Rehabilitation Journal 22(1):55–61, 1998

59. Test MA, Allness DJ, Knoedler WH: Impact of seven years of assertive community treatment. Presented at the American Psychiatric Association Institute on Psychiatric Services, Boston, Oct 6–10, 1995

60. Drake RE, Becker DR, Xie H, et al: Barriers in the brokered model of supported employment for persons with psychiatric disabilities. Journal of Vocational Rehabilitation 5:141–150, 1995

61. Goldberg RW, Lucksted A, McNary S, et al: Correlates of long-term unemployment among inner-city adults with serious and persistent mental illness. Psychiatric Services 52:101–103, 2001

62. Meisler N, Blankertz L, Santos AB, et al: Impact of assertive community treatment on homeless persons with co-occurring severe psychiatric and substance use disorders. Community Mental Health Journal 33:113–122, 1997

63. Sengupta A, Drake RE, McHugo GJ: The relationship between substance use disorder and vocational functioning among persons with severe mental illness. Psychiatric Rehabilitation Journal 22(1):41–45, 1998

64. Alverson H, Vicente E: An ethnographic study of vocational rehabilitation for Puerto Rican Americans with severe mental illness. Psychiatric Rehabilitation Journal 22(1):69–72, 1998

65. Harris M, Bebout RR, Freeman DW, et al: Work stories: psychological responses to work in a population of dually diagnosed adults. Psychiatric Quarterly 68:131–153, 1997

66. Quimby E, Drake RE, Becker DR: Ethnographic findings from the Washington, DC, Vocational Services Study. Psychiatric Rehabilitation Journal, in press

67. Bebout RR, Becker DR, Drake RE: A research induction group for clients entering a mental health research project: a replication study. Community Mental Health Journal 34:289–295, 1998

68. Drake RE, Becker DR, Anthony WA: The use of a research induction group in mental health services research. Hospital and Community Psychiatry 45:487–489, 1994

69. Catalano R, Drake RE, Becker DR, et al: Labor market conditions and employment of the mentally ill. Journal of Mental Health Policy and Economics 2:51–54, 1999

70. Gowdy EA, Rapp CA, Coffman M, et al: The relationship between economic conditions and employment of people with severe and persistent mental illness. Lawrence, University of Kansas, School of Social Welfare, 2000

71. Purlee GD: Predictors of Employment Outcome for Persons With Serious Mental Illness. Ph.D. dissertation. Bloomington, Indiana University, School of Education, 1993

72. Baron R, Salzer MS: The career patterns of persons with serious mental illness: generating a new vision of lifetime careers for those in recovery. Psychiatric Rehabilitation Skills 4:136–156, 2000

73. Adams-Shollenberger GE, Mitchell TE: A comparison of janitorial workers with mental retardation and their non-disabled peers on retention and absenteeism. Journal of Rehabilitation 62(3):56–60, 1996

74. Averett S, Warner R, Little J, et al: Labor supply, disability benefits, and mental illness. Eastern Economic Journal 25:279–288, 1999

75. Rogers ES, MacDonald-Wilson K, Danley K, et al: A process analysis of supported employment services for persons with serious psychiatric disability: implications for program design. Journal of Vocational Rehabilitation 8:233–242, 1997

76. Rollins AL, Bond GR, Salyers MP: Interpersonal relationships on the job: does the employment program make a difference? Presented at the Fourth Biennial Research Seminar on Work, Matrix Research Institute, Philadelphia, Oct 11–13, 2000

77. Bond GR, Meyer PS: The role of medications in the employment of people with schizophrenia. Journal of Rehabilitation 65(4):9–16, 1999

78. Mueser KT, Salyers MP, Mueser PR: A prospective analysis of work in schizophrenia. Schizophrenia Bulletin, in press

79. Rogers ES, Walsh D, Masotta L, et al: Massachusetts Survey of Client Preferences for Community Support Services (final report). Boston, Boston University, Center for Psychiatric Rehabilitation, 1991

80. Anthony WA, Blanch A: Supported employment for persons who are psychiatrically disabled: an historical and conceptual perspective. Psychosocial Rehabilitation Journal 11(2):5–23, 1987

81. Henry GT: Practical Sampling. Newbury Park, Calif, Sage, 1990

82. Hogan MF: Supported Employment: How Can Mental Health Leaders Make a Difference? Columbus, Ohio Department of Mental Health, 1999

83. Bedell JR, Draving D, Parrish A, et al: A description and comparison of experiences of people with mental disorders in supported employment and paid prevocational training. Psychiatric Rehabilitation Journal 21(3):279–283, 1998

84. Hatfield AB: Serving the unserved in community rehabilitation programs. Psychosocial Rehabilitation Journal 13(2):71–82, 1989

85. Hollingsworth EJ, Sweeney JK: Mental health expenditures for services for people with severe mental illness. Psychiatric Services 48:485–490, 1997

86. Leff HS, Wise M: Measuring service system implementation in a public mental health system through provider descriptions of employment service need and use. Psychosocial Rehabilitation Journal 18(4):51–64, 1995

87. Five State Feasibility Study on State Mental Health Agency Performance Measures: Draft Executive Summary. Alexandria, Va, National Association of State Mental Health Program Directors Research Institute, Inc, 1998

88. Wehman P, Moon MS: Vocational Rehabilitation and Supported Employment. Baltimore, Brookes, 1988

89. Noble JH, Honberg RS, Hall LL, et al: A Legacy of Failure: The Inability of the Federal-State Vocational Rehabilitation System to Serve People With Severe Mental Illness. Arlington, Va, National Alliance for the Mentally Ill, 1997

90. Marshak LE, Bostick D, Turton LJ: Closure outcomes for clients with psychiatric disabilities served by the vocational rehabilitation system. Rehabilitation Counseling Bulletin 33:247–250, 1990

91. Wehman P, Revell G: Supported employment: a decade of rapid growth and impact. American Rehabilitation 24(1):31–43, 1998

92. Riggs RT: HMOs and the seriously mentally ill: a view from the trenches. Community Mental Health Journal 32:213–218, 1996

93. Baron RC, Rutman ID, Hadley T: Rehabilitation services for people with long-term mental illness in the managed behavioral health care system: stepchild again? Psychiatric Rehabilitation Journal 20(2):33–38, 1996

94. Vogler KM: A Fidelity Study of the Indiana Supported Employment Model for Individuals With Severe Mental Illness. Ph.D. dissertation. Indianapolis, Indiana University–Purdue University Indianapolis, Department of Psychology, 1998

95. Barton R: Psychosocial rehabilitation services in community support systems: a review of outcomes and policy recommendations. Psychiatric Services 50:525–534, 1999

96. McDonnell J, Nofs D, Hardman M, et al: An analysis of the procedural components of supported employment programs associated with employment outcomes. Journal of Applied Behavior Analysis 22:417–428, 1989

97. Braitman A, Counts P, Davenport R, et al: Comparison of barriers to employment for unemployed and employed clients in a case management program: an exploratory study. Psychiatric Rehabilitation Journal 19(1):3–18, 1995

98. Crane-Ross D, Roth D, Lauber BG: Consumers' and case managers' perceptions of mental health and community support service needs. Community Mental Health Journal 36:161–178, 2000

99. Spaniol L, Jung H, Zipple AM, et al: Families as a resource in the rehabilitation of the severely psychiatrically disabled, in Families of the Mentally Ill: Coping and Adaptation. Edited by Hatfield AB, Lefley HP. New York, Guilford, 1987

100. Gill KJ, Pratt CW, Barrett N: Preparing psychiatric rehabilitation specialists through undergraduate education. Community Mental Health Journal 33:323–329, 1997

101. Noble JH: The benefits and costs of supported employment for people with mental illness and with traumatic brain injury in New York State. Buffalo, Research Foundation of the State University of New York, 1991

102. Shafer MS, Pardee R, Stewart M: An assessment of the training needs of rehabilitation and community mental health workers in a six-state region. Psychiatric Rehabilitation Journal 23(2):161–169, 1999

103. Corrigan PW, McCracken SG: Interactive Staff Training: Rehabilitation Teams That Work. New York, Plenum, 1997

104. Addiction Technology Transfer Center: The Change Book: A Blueprint for Technology Transfer. Rockville, Md, Addiction Technology Transfer Center National Network, 2000

105. Torrey WC, Drake RE, Dixon L, et al: Implementing evidence-based practices for persons with severe mental illness. Psychiatric Services 52:45–50, 2001

106. McCarthy D, Thompson D, Olson S: Planning a statewide project to convert day treatment to supported employment. Psychiatric Rehabilitation Journal 22(1):30–33, 1998

107. Golden TP, O'Mara S, Ferrell C, et al: A theoretical construct for benefits planning and assistance, in the Ticket to Work and Work Incentive Improvement Act. Journal of Vocational Rehabilitation 14:147–152, 2000

108. Brooke V, Green H, O'Brien D, et al: Supported employment: it's working in Alabama. Journal of Vocational Rehabilitation 14:163–171, 2000

109. Novak J, Mank D, Revell G, et al: Paying for success: results-based approaches to funding supported employment, in Supported Employment in Business: Expanding the Capacity of Workers With Disabilities. Edited by Wehman P. St Augustine, Fla, Training Resource Network, in press

110. Bridging Science and Service: A Report by the National Advisory Mental Health Council's Clinical Treatment and Services Research Workgroup. Rockville, Md, National Institute of Mental Health, 1999

111. Position statement on employment and rehabilitation for persons with severe psychiatric disabilities. National Association of State Mental Health Program Directors, 1996. Available at www.nasmhpd.org/employps.htm

112. Batalden PB, Stoltz PK: A framework for the continual improvement of health care: building and applying professional and improvement knowledge to test changes in daily work. Joint Commission 19:424–435, 1993

113. Becker DR, Torrey WC, Toscano R, et al: Building recovery-oriented services: lessons from implementing individual placement and support (IPS) in community mental health centers. Psychiatric Rehabilitation Journal 22(1):51–61, 1998

114. Mank D: The underachievement of supported employment: a call for reinvestment. Journal of Disability Policy Studies 5(2):1–24, 1994

115. Torrey WC, Mead S, Ross G: Addressing the social needs of mental health consumers when day treatment programs convert to supported employment: can consumer-run services play a role? Psychiatric Rehabilitation Journal 22(1):73–75, 1998

116. Bond GR, Evans L, Salyers MP, et al: Measurement of fidelity in psychiatric rehabilitation. Mental Health Services Research 2:75–87, 2000

117. Bond GR, Becker DR, Drake RE, et al: A fidelity scale for the individual placement and support model of supported employment. Rehabilitation Counseling Bulletin 40:265–284, 1997. Instrument available at www.vcu.edu/rrtcweb/sec/outcomes.html

118. Milne D, Gorenski O, Westerman C, e What does it take to transfer training? Psychiatric Rehabilitation Skills 4:259–281, 2000

119. Rapp C, Poertner J: Social Admini tion: A Client-Centered Approach. White Plains, NY, Longman, 1992

120. Backer T, Liberman R, Kuehnel T: semination and adoption of innovative psychosocial interventions. Journal of Consulting and Clinical Psychology 54:111–118, 1986

121. Steinwachs DM, Kasper JD, Skinner Family Perspectives on Meeting the Needs for Care of Severely Mentally Ill Relatives: A National Survey. Baltimore, Johns Hopkins University, Center on the Organization and Financing of Care for the Severely Mentally Ill, 1992

Implementing Dual Diagnosis Services for Clients With Severe Mental Illness

Robert E. Drake, M.D., Ph.D.
Susan M. Essock, Ph.D.
Andrew Shaner, M.D.
Kate B. Carey, Ph.D.
Kenneth Minkoff, M.D.
Lenore Kola, Ph.D.
David Lynde, M.S.W.
Fred C. Osher, M.D.
Robin E. Clark, Ph.D.
Lawrence Rickards, Ph.D.

After 20 years of development and research, dual diagnosis services for clients with severe mental illness are emerging as an evidence-based practice. Effective dual diagnosis programs combine mental health and substance abuse interventions that are tailored for the complex needs of clients with comorbid disorders. The authors describe the critical components of effective programs, which include a comprehensive, long-term, staged approach to recovery; assertive outreach; motivational interventions; provision of help to clients in acquiring skills and supports to manage both illnesses and to pursue functional goals; and cultural sensitivity and competence. Many state mental health systems are implementing dual diagnosis services, but high-quality services are rare. The authors provide an overview of the numerous barriers to implementation and describe implementation strategies to overcome the barriers. Current approaches to implementing dual diagnosis programs involve organizational and financing changes at the policy level, clarity of program mission with structural changes to support dual diagnosis services, training and supervision for clinicians, and dissemination of accurate information to consumers and families to support understanding, demand, and advocacy.

Substance abuse is the most common and clinically significant comorbid disorder among adults with severe mental illness. In this paper the term "substance abuse" refers to substance use disorders, which include abuse and dependence. "Severe mental illness" refers to long-term psychiatric disorders, such as schizophrenia, that are associated with disability and that fall within the traditional purview of public mental health systems. Finally, the term "dual diagnosis" denotes the co-occurrence of substance abuse and severe mental illness.

There are many populations with dual diagnoses, and there are other common terms for this particular group. Furthermore, dual diagnosis is a misleading term because the individuals in this group are heterogeneous and tend to have multiple impairments rather than just two illnesses. Nevertheless, the term appears consistently in the literature and has acquired some coherence as a referent to particular clients, treatments, programs, and service system issues.

Since the problem of dual diagnosis became clinically apparent in the early 1980s (1,2), researchers have established three basic and consistent findings. First, co-occurrence is common; about 50 percent of individuals with severe mental disorders are affected by substance abuse (3). Second, dual diagnosis is associated with a variety of negative outcomes, including higher rates of relapse (4), hospitalization (5), violence (6), incarceration (7), homelessness (8), and serious infections such as HIV and hepatitis (9). Third, the parallel but separate mental health and substance abuse treatment systems so common in the United States deliver fragmented and ineffective care (10). Most clients are unable to navigate the separate systems or make sense of disparate mes-

Dr. Drake and Dr. Clark are affiliated with the New Hampshire–Dartmouth Psychiatric Research Center, 2 Whipple Place, Lebanon, New Hampshire 03766 (e-mail, robert.e.drake@dartmouth.edu). Dr. Essock is with Mt. Sinai Medical School in New York City. Dr. Shaner is affiliated with the School of Medicine at the University of California, Los Angeles. Dr. Carey is with Syracuse University in New York. Dr. Minkoff is in private practice in Boston. Dr. Kola is with Case Western Reserve University in Cleveland, Ohio. Mr. Lynde is with West Institute in Concord, New Hampshire. Dr. Osher is with the University of Maryland School of Medicine in Baltimore. Dr. Rickards is with the Center for Mental Health Services in Rockville, Maryland. This article was originally published in the April 2001 issue of Psychiatric Services.

sages about treatment and recovery. Often they are excluded or extruded from services in one system because of the comorbid disorder and told to return when the other problem is under control. For those reasons, clinicians, administrators, researchers, family organizations, and clients themselves have been calling for the integration of mental health and substance abuse services for at least 15 years (10,11).

Over that time, integrated dual diagnosis services—that is, treatments and programs—have been steadily developed, refined, and evaluated (11). This paper, part of a series on specific evidence-based practices for persons with severe mental illness, provides an overview of the evolution of dual diagnosis services, the evidence on outcomes and critical components, and the limitations of current research. We also address barriers to the implementation of dual diagnosis services and current strategies for implementation in routine mental health settings.

Dual diagnosis services

Treatments, or interventions, are offered within programs that are part of service systems. Dual diagnosis treatments combine or integrate mental health and substance abuse interventions at the level of the clinical interaction. Hence integrated treatment means that the same clinicians or teams of clinicians, working in one setting, provide appropriate mental health and substance abuse interventions in a coordinated fashion. In other words, the caregivers take responsibility for combining the interventions into one coherent package. For the individual with a dual diagnosis, the services appear seamless, with a consistent approach, philosophy, and set of recommendations. The need to negotiate with separate clinical teams, programs, or systems disappears.

Integration involves not only combining appropriate treatments for both disorders but also modifying traditional interventions (12–15). For example, social skills training emphasizes the importance of developing relationships but also the need to avoid social situations that could lead to substance use. Substance abuse

counseling goes slowly, in accordance with the cognitive deficits, negative symptoms, vulnerability to confrontation, and greater need for support that are characteristic of many individuals with severe mental illness. Family interventions address understanding and learning to cope with two interacting illnesses.

The goal of dual diagnosis interventions is recovery from two serious illnesses (16). In this context, "recovery" means that the individual with a dual diagnosis learns to manage both illnesses so that he or she can pursue meaningful life goals (17,18).

Research on dual diagnosis practices

In most states, the publicly financed mental health system bears responsibility for providing treatments and support services for clients with severe mental illness. Dual diagnosis treatments for these clients have therefore generally been added to community support programs within the mental health system.

Early studies of dual diagnosis interventions during the 1980s examined the application of traditional substance abuse treatments, such as 12-step groups, to clients with mental disorders within mental health programs. These studies had disappointing results for at least two reasons (19). The clinical programs did not take into account the complex needs of the population, and researchers had not yet solved basic methodologic problems. For example, early programs often failed to incorporate outreach and motivational interventions, and evaluations were limited by lack of reliable and valid assessment of substance abuse. Reviews based on these early studies were understandably pessimistic (20).

At the same time, however, a series of demonstration projects using more comprehensive programs that incorporated assertive outreach and long-term rehabilitation began to show better outcomes. Moreover, the projects developed motivational interventions to help clients who did not perceive or acknowledge their substance abuse or mental illness problems (21).

Building on these insights, projects in the early 1990s incorporated moti-

vational approaches as well as outreach, comprehensiveness, and a long-term perspective, often within the structure of multidisciplinary treatment teams. These later studies, which were uncontrolled but incorporated more valid measures of substance abuse, generally showed positive outcomes, including substantial rates of stable remission of substance abuse (22–25). Of course, uncontrolled studies of this type often produce findings that are not replicated in controlled studies; they should be considered pilot studies, which are often needed to refine the intervention and the methodologies of evaluation and which should be followed by controlled investigation to determine evidence-based practice (26).

Controlled research studies of comprehensive dual diagnosis programs began to appear in the mid-1990s. Eight recent studies with experimental or quasi-experimental designs support the effectiveness of integrated dual diagnosis treatments for clients with severe mental illness and substance use disorders (27–34). The type and array of dual diagnosis interventions in these programs vary, but they include several common components, which are reviewed below. The eight studies demonstrated a variety of positive outcomes in domains such as substance abuse, psychiatric symptoms, housing, hospitalization, arrests, functional status, and quality of life (19). Although each had methodological limitations, together they indicate that current integrated treatment programs are more effective than nonintegrated programs. By contrast, the evidence continues to show that dual diagnosis clients in mental health programs that fail to integrate substance abuse interventions have poor outcomes (35).

Critical components

Several components of integrated programs can be considered evidence-based practices because they are almost always present in programs that have demonstrated good outcomes in controlled studies and because their absence is associated with predictable failures (21). For example, dual diagnosis programs that include assertive outreach are able to engage and retain clients at a high rate, while those that fail to include outreach lose many clients.

Staged interventions

Effective programs incorporate, implicitly or explicitly, the concept of stages of treatment (14,36,37). In the simplest conceptualization, stages of treatment include forming a trusting relationship (engagement), helping the engaged client develop the motivation to become involved in recovery-oriented interventions (persuasion), helping the motivated client acquire skills and supports for controlling illnesses and pursuing goals (active treatment), and helping the client in stable remission develop and use strategies for maintaining recovery (relapse prevention).

Clients do not move linearly through stages. They sometimes enter services at advanced levels, skip over or pass rapidly through stages, or relapse to earlier stages. They may be in different stages with respect to mental illness and substance abuse. Nevertheless, the concept of stages has proved useful to program planners and clinicians because clients at different stages respond to stage-specific interventions.

Assertive outreach

Many clients with a dual diagnosis have difficulty linking with services and participating in treatment (38). Effective programs engage clients and members of their support systems by providing assertive outreach, usually through some combination of intensive case management and meetings in the client's residence (21,32). For example, homeless persons with dual diagnoses often benefit from outreach, help with housing, and time to develop a trusting relationship before participating in any formal treatment. These approaches enable clients to gain access to services and maintain needed relationships with a consistent program over months and years. Without such efforts, noncompliance and dropout rates are high (39).

Motivational interventions

Most dual diagnosis clients have little readiness for abstinence-oriented treatment (40,41). Many also lack motivation to manage psychiatric illness and to pursue employment or other functional goals. Effective programs therefore incorporate motivational interventions that are designed to help clients become ready for more definitive interventions aimed at illness self-management (12,14,21). For example, clients who are so demoralized, symptomatic, or confused that they mistakenly believe that alcohol and cocaine are helping them to cope better than medications require education, support, and counseling to develop hope and a realistic understanding of illnesses, drugs, treatments, and goals.

Motivational interventions involve helping the individual identify his or her own goals and to recognize, through a systematic examination of the individual's ambivalence, that not managing one's illnesses interferes with attaining those goals (42). Recent research has demonstrated that clients who are not motivated can be reliably identified (43) and effectively helped with motivational interventions (Carey KB, Carey MP, Maisto SA, et al, unpublished data, 2000).

Counseling

Once clients are motivated to manage their own illnesses, they need to develop skills and supports to control symptoms and to pursue an abstinent lifestyle. Effective programs provide some form of counseling that promotes cognitive and behavioral skills at this stage. The counseling takes different forms and formats, such as group, individual, or family therapy or a combination (15). Few studies have compared specific approaches to counseling, although one study did find preliminary evidence that a cognitive-behavioral approach was superior to a 12-step approach (28). At least three research groups are actively working to refine cognitive-behavioral approaches to substance abuse counseling for dual diagnosis clients (12,13,44). These approaches often incorporate motivational sessions at the beginning of counseling and as needed in subsequent sessions rather than as separate interventions.

Social support interventions

In addition to helping clients build skills for managing their illness and pursuing goals, effective programs focus on strengthening the immediate social environment to help them modify their behavior. These activities, which recognize the role of social networks in recovery from dual disorders (45), include social network or family interventions.

Long-term perspective

Effective programs recognize that recovery tends to occur over months or years in the community. People with severe mental illness and substance abuse do not usually develop stability and functional improvements quickly, even in intensive treatment programs, unless they enter treatment at an advanced stage (19). Instead, they tend to improve over months and years in conjunction with a consistent dual diagnosis program. Effective programs therefore take a long-term, community-based perspective that includes rehabilitation activities to prevent relapses and to enhance gains.

Comprehensiveness

Learning to lead a symptom-free, abstinent lifestyle that is satisfying and sustainable often requires transforming many aspects of one's life—for example, habits, stress management, friends, activities, and housing. Therefore, in effective programs attention to substance abuse as well as mental illness is integrated into all aspects of the existing mental health program and service system rather than isolated as a discrete substance abuse treatment intervention. Inpatient hospitalization, assessment, crisis intervention, medication management, money management, laboratory screening, housing, and vocational rehabilitation incorporate special features that are tailored specifically for dual diagnosis patients. For example, hospitalization is considered a component of the system that supports movement toward recovery by providing diagnosis, stabilization, and linkage with outpatient dual diagnosis interventions during acute episodes (46). Similarly, housing and vocational programs can be used to support the individual with a dual diagnosis in acquiring skills and supports needed for recovery (47).

*Cultural sensitivity
and competence*

A fundamental finding of the demonstration programs of the late 1980s was that cultural sensitivity and competence were critical to engaging clients in dual diagnosis services (21). These demonstrations showed that African Americans, Hispanics, and other underserved groups, such as farm workers, homeless persons, women with children, inner-city residents, and persons in rural areas, could be engaged in dual diagnosis services if the services were tailored to their particular racial, cultural, and other group characteristics.

Many dual diagnosis programs omit some of these critical components as evidence-based practices. However, one consistent finding in the research is that programs that show high fidelity to the model described here—those that incorporate more of the core elements—produce better outcomes than low-fidelity programs (32,48,49). A common misconception about technology transfer is that model programs are not generalizable and that local solutions are superior. A more accurate reading of the research is that modifications for cultural and other local circumstances are important, but critical program components must be replicated to achieve good outcomes.

Limitations of the research

The design and quality of research procedures and data across dual diagnosis studies are inconsistent. In addition, researchers have thus far failed to address a number of issues.

Dual diagnosis research has studied the clinical enterprise, that is, treatments and programs, with little attention to the policy or system perspective. Despite widespread endorsement of integrated dual diagnosis services (13,50–53), there continues to be a general failure at the federal and state levels to resolve problems related to organization and financing (see below). Thus, despite the emergence of many excellent programs around the country, few if any large mental health systems have been able to accomplish widespread implementation of dual diagnosis services for persons with severe mental illness.

We are aware of no specific studies of strategies to finance, contract for, reorganize, or train in relation to dual diagnosis services.

Lack of data on the cost of integrated dual diagnosis services and the cost savings of providing good care impedes policy development. Dual diagnosis clients incur high treatment costs in usual services (54,55), and care is costly to their families (56), but effective treatment may be even more costly. Some studies suggest cost savings related to providing good services (57,58), but these are not definitive.

Another limitation of the research is the lack of specificity of dual diagnosis treatments. Interventions differ across studies, manuals and fidelity measures are rare, and no consensus exists on specific approaches to individual counseling, group treatment, family intervention, housing, medications, and other components. Current research will address some of these issues by refining specific components, although efficacy studies may identify complex and expensive interventions that will be impractical in routine mental health settings.

A majority of dual diagnosis clients respond well to integrated outpatient services, but clients who do not respond continue to be at high risk of hospitalization, incarceration, homelessness, HIV infection, and other serious adverse outcomes. Other than one study of long-term residential treatment (33), controlled research has not addressed clients who do not respond to outpatient services. Other potential interventions include outpatient commitment (59), treatments aimed at trauma sequelae (60), money management (61), contingency management (62), and pharmacological approaches using medications such as clozapine (63), disulfiram (64), or naltrexone.

Although a few studies have explored the specific treatment needs of dual diagnosis clients who are women (65,66) or minorities (21,67), particular program modifications for these groups need further validation. For example, many dual diagnosis programs have identified high rates of trauma histories and sequelae among women (46,68,69), and studies have

suggested interventions to address trauma; however, no data on outcomes are yet available.

Implementation barriers

Although integrated dual diagnosis services and other evidence-based practices are widely advocated, they are rarely offered in routine mental health treatment settings (70). The barriers are legion.

Policy barriers

State, county, and city mental health authorities often encounter policies related to organizational structure, financing, regulations, and licensing that militate against the functional integration of mental health and substance abuse services (71). The U.S. public mental health and substance abuse treatment systems grew independently. In most states these services are provided under the auspices of separate cabinet-level departments with separate funding streams, advocacy groups, lobbyists, enabling legislation, information systems, job classifications, and criteria for credentials. Huge fiscal incentives and strong political allies act to maintain the status quo.

Medicaid programs, which fund a significant and growing proportion of treatment for persons with severe mental illness, vary substantially from state to state in the types of mental health and substance abuse services they fund. In most states, mental health and substance abuse agencies have little control over how Medicaid services are reimbursed or administered, which makes it difficult for public systems to ensure that appropriate services are accessible. Medicare, the federal insurance program for elderly and disabled persons, generally pays for a more limited scope of mental health and substance abuse services. Together Medicaid and Medicare pay for more than 30 percent of all behavioral health services, but their impact on dual diagnosis services has not been studied (72).

Program barriers

At the local level, administrators of clinics, centers, and programs have often lacked the clear service models, administrative guidelines, contractual incentives, quality assurance procedures, and outcome measures needed to implement dual diagnosis services. When clinical needs compel them to move ahead anyway, they have difficulty hiring a skilled workforce with experience in providing dual diagnosis interventions and lack the resources to train current supervisors and clinicians.

Clinical barriers

The beliefs of the mental health and substance abuse treatment traditions are inculcated in clinicians, which diminishes the opportunities for cross-fertilization (73). Although an integrated clinical philosophy and a practical approach to dual diagnosis treatment have been clearly delineated for more than a decade (16), educational institutions rarely teach this approach. Consequently, mental health clinicians typically lack training in dual diagnosis treatment and have to rely on informal, self-initiated opportunities for learning current interventions (74). They often avoid diagnosing substance abuse when they believe that it is irrelevant, that it will interfere with funding, or that they cannot treat it. Clinicians trained in substance abuse treatment, as well as recovering dual diagnosis clients, could add expertise and training, but they are often excluded from jobs in the mental health system.

Consumer and family barriers

Clients and their families rarely have good information about dual diagnosis and appropriate services. Few programs offer psychoeducational services related to dual diagnosis, although practical help from families plays a critical role in recovery (75). Family members are often unaware of substance abuse, blame all symptoms on drug abuse, or attribute symptoms and substance use to willful misbehavior. Supporting family involvement is an important but neglected role for clinicians.

Consumers often deny or minimize problems related to substance abuse (40) and, like other substance abusers, believe that alcohol or other drugs are helpful in alleviating distress. They may be legitimately con-

fused about causality because they perceive the immediate effects of drugs rather than the intermediate or long-term consequences (76). The net result is that the individual lacks motivation to pursue active substance abuse treatment, which can reinforce clinical inattention.

Implementation strategies

There are no proven strategies for overcoming the aforementioned barriers to implementing dual diagnosis services, but some suggestions have come from systems and programs that have had moderate success.

Recent research offers evidence that integrated dual diagnosis treatments are effective, but basic interventions are rarely incorporated into the mental health programs in which these clients receive care.

Policy strategies

Health care authorities in a majority of, and possibly all, states have current initiatives for creating dual diagnosis services. Because health care policy is often administered at the county or city level, hundreds of individual experiments are occurring. One initial branch point involves the decision to focus broadly on the entire behavioral health system—that is, on all clients with mental health and substance abuse problems—or more narrowly on services for those with

severe mental illness and co-occurring substance abuse. We examine here only strategies for dual diagnosis clients with severe mental illness, for whom the implementation issues are relatively distinct.

Commonly used system-level strategies include building a consensus around the vision for integrated services and then conjointly planning; specifying a model; implementing structural, regulatory, and reimbursement changes; establishing contracting mechanisms; defining standards; and funding demonstration programs and training initiatives (77). To our knowledge, few efforts have been made to study these efforts at the system level.

Anecdotal evidence indicates that blending mental health and substance abuse funds appears to have been a relatively unsuccessful strategy, especially early in the course of system change. Fear of losing money to cover nontraditional populations often leads to prolonged disagreements, inability to develop consensus, and abandonment of other plans. As a less controversial, preliminary step, the mental health authority often assumes responsibility for comprehensive care, including substance abuse treatment, for persons with severe mental illness, while the substance abuse authority assists by pledging to help with training and planning.

This limited approach enables the mental health system to attract and train dual diagnosis specialists who can subsequently train other clinicians and programs. Without structural, regulatory, and funding changes to reinforce the training, however, the expertise may soon disappear—a common experience after demonstration projects. Thus many experts advise that policy issues should be addressed early in the process of implementation to avoid wasting efforts on training (78–80).

New costs to the mental health system for dual diagnosis training could be offset by greater effectiveness in ameliorating substance-abusing behaviors that are associated with hospitalizations. However, saving costs over time assumes that providers are at risk for all treatment costs, that is, that providers have incentives to invest more in outpatient services in order to spend less on inpatient services. Despite the growth of managed care, providers rarely bear complete financial responsibility for the treatment of clients with severe mental illness.

Program strategies

At the level of the mental health clinic or program leadership, the fundamental task is to begin recognizing and treating substance abuse rather than ignoring it or using it as a criterion for exclusion (81). After consensus-building activities to prepare for change, staff need training and supervision to learn new skills, and they must receive reinforcement for acquiring and using these skills effectively. One common strategy is to appoint a director of dual diagnosis services whose job is to plan and oversee the training of staff, the integration of substance abuse awareness and treatment into all aspects of the mental health program, and the monitoring and reinforcement of these activities through medical records, quality assurance activities, and outcome data.

Experts identify the importance of having a single leader for program change (82). Fidelity measures for integrated dual diagnosis services can facilitate successful implementation at the program level (50,83). Monitoring and reinforcing mechanisms also emphasize client-centered outcomes, such as abstinence and employment.

Clinical strategies

Mental health clinicians need to acquire knowledge and a core set of skills related to substance abuse that includes assessing substance abuse, providing motivational interventions for clients who are not ready to participate in abstinence-oriented treatment, and providing counseling for those who are motivated try to maintain abstinence. Clinicians adopt new skills as a result of motivation, instruction, practice, and reinforcement (84). Because substance abuse affects the lives of the great majority of clients with severe mental illness—as a co-occurring disorder, family stressor, or environmental hazard—all clinicians

should learn these basic skills. Otherwise substance abuse problems will continue to be missed and untreated in this population (85,86).

For example, all case managers should recognize and address substance abuse in their daily interactions, as should housing staff, employment specialists, and other staff. Until professional educational programs begin teaching current dual diagnosis treatment techniques (87), mental health system leaders will bear the burden of training staff.

Some staff will become dual diagnosis specialists and acquire more than the basic skills. These individuals will be counted on to lead dual diagnosis groups, family interventions, residential programs, and other specialized services.

Consumer- and family-level strategies

Clients and family members need access to accurate information. Otherwise their opportunities to make informed choices, to request effective services, and to advocate for system changes are severely compromised. Consumer demand and family advocacy can move the health care system toward evidence-based practices, but concerted efforts at the national, state, and local levels are required. Researchers can facilitate their efforts by offering clear messages about the forms, processes, and expected outcomes of evidence-based practices. Similarly, local programs should provide information on available dual diagnosis services to clients and their families.

As consumers move into roles as providers within the mental health system and in consumer-run services, they also need training in dual diagnosis treatments. Local educational programs, such as community colleges, as well as staff training programs should address these needs.

Conclusions

Substance abuse is a common and devastating comorbid disorder among persons with severe mental illness. Recent research offers evidence that integrated dual diagnosis treatments are effective, but basic interventions are rarely incorporated into the men-

tal health programs in which these clients receive care. Successful implementation of dual diagnosis services within mental health systems will depend on changes at several levels: clear policy directives with consistent organizational and financing supports, program changes to incorporate the mission of addressing co-occurring substance abuse, supports for the acquisition of expertise at the clinical level, and availability of accurate information to consumers and family members. ◆

Acknowledgments

This review by a national panel was supported by grant 036805 from the Robert Wood Johnson Foundation and contract 280-00-8049 from the Center for Mental Health Services.

References

1. Pepper B, Krishner MC, Ryglewicz H: The young adult chronic patient: overview of a population. Hospital and Community Psychiatry 32:463–469, 1981

2. Caton CLM: The new chronic patient and the system of community care. Hospital and Community Psychiatry 32:475–478, 1981

3. Regier DA, Farmer ME, Rae DS, et al: Comorbidity of mental disorders with alcohol and other drug abuse. JAMA 264:2511–2518, 1990

4. Swofford C, Kasckow J, Scheller-Gilkey G, et al: Substance use: a powerful predictor of relapse in schizophrenia. Schizophrenia Research 20:145–151, 1996

5. Haywood TW, Kravitz HM, Grossman LS, et al: Predicting the "revolving door" phenomenon among patients with schizophrenic, schizoaffective, and affective disorders. American Journal of Psychiatry 152:856–861, 1995

6. Cuffel B, Shumway M, Chouljian T: A longitudinal study of substance use and community violence in schizophrenia. Journal of Nervous and Mental Disease 182:704–708, 1994

7. Abram KM, Teplin LA: Co-occurring disorders among mentally ill jail detainees: implications for public policy. American Psychologist 46:1036–1045, 1991

8. Caton CLM, Shrout PE, Eagle PF, et al: Risk factors for homelessness among schizophrenic men: a case-control study. American Journal of Public Health 84:265–270, 1994

9. Rosenberg SD, Goodman LA, Osher FC, et al: Prevalence of HIV, hepatitis B, and hepatitis C in people with severe mental illness. American Journal of Public Health 91:31–37, 2001

10. Ridgely MS, Osher FC, Goldman HH, et

al: Executive Summary: Chronic Mentally Ill Young Adults With Substance Abuse Problems: A Review of Research, Treatment, and Training Issues. Baltimore, University of Maryland School of Medicine, Mental Health Services Research Center, 1987

11. Drake RE, Wallach MA: Dual diagnosis: 15 years of progress. Psychiatric Services 51:1126–1129, 2000

12. Barrowclough C, Haddock G, Tarrier N, et al: Cognitive-behavioral intervention for clients with severe mental illness who have a substance misuse problem. Psychiatric Rehabilitation Skills 4:216–233, 2000

13. Bellack AS, DiClemente CC: Treating substance abuse among patients with schizophrenia. Psychiatric Services 50:75–80, 1999

14. Carey KB: Substance use reduction in the context of outpatient psychiatric treatment: a collaborative, motivational, harm reduction approach. Community Mental Health Journal 32:291–306, 1996

15. Mueser KT, Drake RE, Noordsy DL: Integrated mental health and substance abuse treatment for severe psychiatric disorders. Journal of Practical Psychiatry and Behavioral Health 4:129–139, 1998

16. Minkoff K: An integrated treatment model for dual diagnosis of psychosis and addiction. Hospital and Community Psychiatry 40:1031–1036, 1989

17. Mead S, Copeland ME: What recovery means to us: consumers' perspectives. Community Mental Health Journal 36:315–328, 2000

18. Torrey WC, Wyzik P: The recovery vision as a service improvement guide for community mental health center providers. Community Mental Health Journal 36:209–216, 2000

19. Drake RE, Mercer-McFadden C, Mueser KT, et al: Review of integrated mental health and substance abuse treatment for patients with dual disorders. Schizophrenia Bulletin 24:589–608, 1998

20. Ley A, Jeffery DP, McLaren S, et al: Treatment programmes for people with both severe mental illness and substance misuse. Cochrane Library, Feb 1999. Available at http://www.update-software.com/cochrane/cochrane-frame.html

21. Mercer-McFadden C, Drake RE, Brown NB, et al: The community support program demonstrations of services for young adults with severe mental illness and substance use disorders, 1987–1991. Psychiatric Rehabilitation Journal 20(3):13–24, 1997

22. Detrick A, Stiepock V: Treating persons with mental illness, substance abuse, and legal problems: the Rhode Island experience. New Directions for Mental Health Services, no 56:65–77, 1992

23. Drake RE, McHugo G, Noordsy DL: Treatment of alcoholism among schizophrenic outpatients: four-year outcomes. American Journal of Psychiatry 150:328–329, 1993

24. Durell J, Lechtenberg B, Corse S, et al: Intensive case management of persons with chronic mental illness who abuse substances. Hospital and Community Psychiatry 44:415–416, 1993

25. Meisler N, Blankertz L, Santos AB, et al: Impact of assertive community treatment on homeless persons with co-occurring severe psychiatric and substance use disorders. Community Mental Health Journal 33:113–122, 1997

26. Drake RE, Goldman HH, Leff HS, et al: Implementing evidence-based practices in routine mental health service settings. Psychiatric Services 52:179–182, 2001

27. Godley SH, Hoewing-Roberson R, Godley MD: Final MISA Report. Bloomington, Ill, Lighthouse Institute, 1994

28. Jerrell JM, Ridgely MS: Comparative effectiveness of three approaches to serving people with severe mental illness and substance abuse disorders. Journal of Nervous and Mental Disease 183:566–576, 1995

29. Drake RE, Yovetich NA, Bebout RR, et al: Integrated treatment for dually diagnosed homeless adults. Journal of Nervous and Mental Disease 185:298–305, 1997

30. Carmichael D, Tackett-Gibson M, Dell O, et al: Texas Dual Diagnosis Project Evaluation Report, 1997–1998. College Station, Tex, Texas A&M University, Public Policy Research Institute, 1998

31. Drake RE, McHugo GJ, Clark RE, et al: Assertive community treatment for patients with co-occurring severe mental illness and substance use disorder: a clinical trial. American Journal of Orthopsychiatry 68:201–215, 1998

32. Ho AP, Tsuang JW, Liberman RP, et al: Achieving effective treatment of patients with chronic psychotic illness and comorbid substance dependence. American Journal of Psychiatry 156:1765–1770, 1999

33. Brunette MF, Drake RE, Woods M, et al: A comparison of long-term and short-term residential treatment programs for dual diagnosis patients. Psychiatric Services 52:526–528, 2001

34. Barrowclough C, Haddock G, Tarrier N, et al: Randomised controlled trial of motivational interviewing and cognitive behavioural intervention for schizophrenia patients with associated drug or alcohol misuse. American Journal of Psychiatry, in press

35. Havassy BE, Shopshire MS, Quigley LA: Effects of substance dependence on outcomes of patients in a randomized trial of two case management models. Psychiatric Services 51:639–644, 2000

36. Osher FC, Kofoed LL: Treatment of patients with psychiatric and psychoactive substance use disorders. Hospital and Community Psychiatry 40:1025–1030, 1989

37. McHugo GJ, Drake RE, Burton HL, et al: A scale for assessing the stage of substance abuse treatment in persons with severe mental illness. Journal of Nervous and Mental Disease 183:762–767, 1995

38. Owen C, Rutherford V, Jones M, et al: Noncompliance in psychiatric aftercare. Community Mental Health Journal 33:25–34, 1997

39. Hellerstein DJ, Rosenthal RN, Miner CR: A prospective study of integrated outpatient treatment for substance-abusing schizophrenic patients. American Journal on Addictions 42:33–42, 1995

40. Test MA, Wallish LS, Allness DG, et al: Substance use in young adults with schizophrenic disorders. Schizophrenia Bulletin 15:465–476, 1989

41. Ziedonis D, Trudeau K: Motivation to quit using substances among individuals with schizophrenia: implications for a motivation-based treatment model. Schizophrenia Bulletin 23:229–238, 1997

42. Miller W, Rollnick S: Motivational Interviewing: Preparing People to Change Addictive Behavior. New York, Guilford, 1991

43. Carey KB, Maisto SA, Carey MP, et al: Measuring readiness-to-change substance misuse among psychiatric outpatients: I. reliability and validity of self-report measures. Journal of Studies on Alcohol, in press

44. Roberts LJ, Shaner A, Eckman T: Overcoming Addictions: Skills Training for People With Schizophrenia. New York, Norton, 1999

45. Alverson H, Alverson M, Drake RE: An ethnographic study of the longitudinal course of substance abuse among people with severe mental illness. Community Mental Health Journal 36:557–569, 2000

46. Greenfield SF, Weiss RD, Tohen M: Substance abuse and the chronically mentally ill: a description of dual diagnosis treatment services in a psychiatric hospital. Community Mental Health Journal 31:265–278, 1995

47. Drake RE, Mueser KT: Psychosocial approaches to dual diagnosis. Schizophrenia Bulletin 26:105–118, 2000

48. Jerrell JM, Ridgely MS: Impact of robustness of program implementation on outcomes of clients in dual diagnosis programs. Psychiatric Services 50:109–112, 1999

49. McHugo GJ, Drake RE, Teague GB, et al: Fidelity to assertive community treatment and client outcomes in the New Hampshire dual disorders study. Psychiatric Services 50:818–824, 1999

50. Rach-Beisel J, Scott J, Dixon L: Co-occurring severe mental illness and substance use disorders: a review of recent research. Psychiatric Services 50:1427–1434, 1999

51. Mueser KT, Bellack A, Blanchard J: Comorbidity of schizophrenia and substance abuse. Journal of Consulting and Clinical Psychology 60:845–856, 1992

52. Osher FC, Drake RE: Reversing a history of unmet needs: approaches to care for persons with co-occurring addictive and mental disorders. American Journal of Orthopsychiatry 66:4–11, 1996

53. Woody G: The challenge of dual diagnosis.

Alcohol Health and Research World 20:76–80, 1996

54. Bartels SJ, Teague GB, Drake RE, et al: Service utilization and costs associated with substance abuse among rural schizophrenic patients. Journal of Nervous and Mental Disease 181:227–232, 1993

55. Dickey B, Azeni H: Persons with dual diagnosis of substance abuse and major mental illness: their excess costs of psychiatric care. American Journal of Public Health 86:973–977, 1996

56. Clark RE: Family costs associated with severe mental illness and substance use. Hospital and Community Psychiatry 45:808–813, 1994

57. Clark RE, Teague GB, Ricketts SK, et al: Cost-effectiveness of assertive community treatment versus standard case management for persons with co-occurring severe mental illness and substance use disorders. Health Services Research 33:1283–1306, 1998

58. Jerrell JM: Cost-effective treatment for persons with dual disorders. New Directions for Mental Health Services, no 70:79–91, 1996

59. O'Keefe C, Potenza DP, Mueser KT: Treatment outcomes for severely mentally ill patients on conditional discharge to community-based treatment. Journal of Nervous and Mental Disease 185:409–411, 1997

60. Harris M: Trauma Recovery and Empowerment Manual. Edited by Anglin J. New York, Free Press, 1998

61. Ries RK, Dyck DG: Representative payee practices of community mental health centers in Washington State. Psychiatric Services 48:811–814, 1997

62. Shaner A, Roberts LJ, Eckman TA, et al: Monetary reinforcement of abstinence from cocaine among mentally ill patients with cocaine dependence. Psychiatric Services 48:807–810, 1997

63. Zimmet SV, Strous RD, Burgess ES, et al: Effects of clozapine on substance use in patients with schizophrenia and schizoaffective disorders: a retrospective survey. Journal of Clinical Psychopharmacology 20:94–98, 2000

64. Mueser KT, Noordsy DL, Essock S: Use of disulfiram in the treatment of patients with dual diagnosis. American Journal of Addiction, in press

65. Brunette MF, Drake RE: Gender differences in patients with schizophrenia and substance abuse. Comprehensive Psychiatry 38:109–116, 1997

66. Alexander MJ: Women with co-occurring addictive and mental disorders: an emerging profile of vulnerability. American Journal of Orthopsychiatry 66:61–70, 1996

67. Quimby E: Homeless clients' perspectives on recovery in the Washington, DC, Dual Diagnosis Project. Contemporary Drug Problems, Summer 1995, pp 265–289

68. Goodman LA, Rosenberg SD, Mueser KT, et al: Physical and sexual assault history in women with serious mental illness: prevalence, correlates, treatment, and future research directions. Schizophrenia Bulletin 23:685–696, 1997

69. Mueser KT, Goodman LB, Trumbetta SL, et al: Trauma and posttraumatic stress disorder in severe mental illness. Journal of Consulting and Clinical Psychology 66:493–499, 1998

70. Surgeon General's Report on Mental Health. Washington, DC, US Government Printing Office, 2000

71. Ridgely M, Goldman H, Willenbring M: Barriers to the care of persons with dual diagnoses: organizational and financing issues. Schizophrenia Bulletin 16:123–132, 1990

72. Mark T, McKusick D, King E, et al: National Expenditures for Mental Health, Alcohol, and Other Drug Abuse Treatment. Rockville, Md, Substance Abuse and Mental Health Services Administration, 1998

73. Drainoni M, Bachman S: Overcoming treatment barriers to providing services for adults with dual diagnosis: three approaches. Journal of Disability Policy Studies 6:43–55, 1995

74. Carey KB, Purnine DM, Maisto SM, et al: Treating substance abuse in the context of severe and persistent mental illness: clinicians' perspectives. Journal of Substance Abuse Treatment 19:189–198, 2000

75. Clark RE: Family support and substance use outcomes for persons with mental illness and substance use disorders. Schizophrenia Bulletin, in press

76. Mueser KT, Drake R, Wallach M: Dual diagnosis: a review of etiological theories. Addictive Behaviors 23:717–734, 1998

77. Co-occurring Psychiatric and Substance Disorders in Managed Care Systems. Rockville, Md, Mental Health Services, 1998

78. Hesketh B: Dilemmas in training for transfer and retention. Applied Psychology 46:317–386, 1997

79. Milne D, Gorenski O, Westerman C, et al: What does it take to transfer training? Psychiatric Rehabilitation Skills 4:259–281, 2000

80. Rapp CA, Poertner J: Social Administration: A Client-Centered Approach. White Plains, NY, Longman, 1992

81. Mercer-McFadden C, Drake RE, Clark RE, et al: Substance Abuse Treatment for People With Severe Mental Disorders. Concord, NH, New Hampshire–Dartmouth Psychiatric Research Center, 1998

82. Corrigan PW: Wanted: champions of rehabilitation for psychiatric hospitals. American Psychologist 40:514–521, 1995

83. Mueser KT, Fox L: Stagewise Family Treatment for Dual Disorders: Treatment Manual. Concord, NH, New Hampshire–Dartmouth Psychiatric Research Center, 1998

84. Torrey WC, Drake RE, Dixon L, et al: Implementing evidence-based practices for persons with severe mental illnesses. Psychiatric Services 52:45–50, 2001

85. Shaner A, Khaka E, Roberts L, et al: Unrecognized cocaine use among schizophrenic patients. American Journal of Psychiatry 150:777–783, 1993

86. Ananth J, Vandewater S, Kamal M, et al: Missed diagnosis of substance abuse in psychiatric patients. Hospital and Community Psychiatry 40:297–299, 1989

87. Carey KB, Bradizza CM, Stasiewicz PR, et al: The case for enhanced addictions training in graduate programs. Behavior Therapist 22:27–31, 1999

Moving Assertive Community Treatment Into Standard Practice

Susan D. Phillips, M.S.W.
Barbara J. Burns, Ph.D.
Elizabeth R. Edgar, M.S.S.W.
Kim T. Mueser, Ph.D.
Karen W. Linkins, Ph.D.
Robert A. Rosenheck, M.D.
Robert E. Drake, M.D., Ph.D.
Elizabeth C. McDonel Herr, Ph.D.

This article describes the assertive community treatment model of comprehensive community-based psychiatric care for persons with severe mental illness and discusses issues pertaining to implementation of the model. The assertive community treatment model has been the subject of more than 25 randomized controlled trials. Research has shown that this type of program is effective in reducing hospitalization, is no more expensive than traditional care, and is more satisfactory to consumers and their families than standard care. Despite evidence of the efficacy of assertive community treatment, it is not uniformly available to the individuals who might benefit from it.

There is mounting interest among mental health care professionals in making mental health practices with demonstrated efficacy and effectiveness available in routine care settings (1,2). One such practice is assertive community treatment, a comprehensive community-based model for delivering treatment, support, and rehabilitation services to individuals with severe mental illness. Assertive community treatment is sometimes referred to as training in community living, the Program for Assertive Community Treatment (PACT), continuous treatment teams, and, within the Department of Veterans Affairs (VA), intensive psychiatric community care.

Assertive community treatment is appropriate for individuals who experience the most intractable symptoms of severe mental illness and the greatest level of functional impairment. These individuals are often heavy users of inpatient psychiatric services, and they frequently have the poorest quality of life.

Research has shown that assertive community treatment is no more expensive than other types of community-based care and that it is more satisfactory to consumers and their families (3). Reviews of the research consistently conclude that compared with other treatments under controlled conditions, such as brokered case management or clinical case management, assertive community treatment results in a greater reduction in psychiatric hospitalization and a higher level of housing stability. The effects of assertive community treatment on quality of life, symptoms, and social functioning are similar to those produced by these other treatments (3–8). Other studies have found associations between assertive community treatment and a lower level of substance use among individuals with dual diagnoses (9,10).

Cost analyses have shown that assertive community treatment is cost-effective for patients with extensive prior hospital use (11–16), and in the long run it may provide a more cost-effective alternative to standard case management for individuals with co-occurring substance use disorders (17). Consumer satisfaction has been less thoroughly investigated; however, the majority of existing studies found that consumers and their fami-

Ms. Phillips is a research associate and Dr. Burns is professor of medical psychology at Duke University Medical Center. Ms. Edgar is director of the National Alliance for the Mentally Ill Technical Assistance Center for the Program for Assertive Community Treatment in Arlington, Virginia. Dr. Linkins is vice-president of the Lewin Group in Falls Church, Virginia. Dr. Rosenheck is director of the Northeast Program Evaluation Center of the Veterans Affairs Connecticut Healthcare in West Haven and professor in the departments of psychiatry and public health at Yale University School of Medicine in New Haven. Dr. Mueser and Dr. Drake are professors at Dartmouth Medical School and scientific director and director, respectively, of the New Hampshire–Dartmouth Psychiatric Research Center. Dr. McDonel Herr is with the Substance Abuse and Mental Health Services Administration in Rockville, Maryland. Address correspondence to Ms. Phillips at Box 3454, Duke University Medical Center, Durham, North Carolina 27710 (e-mail, sphillips@psych.mc.duke.edu). This article was originally published in the June 2001 issue of Psychiatric Services.

lies were more satisfied with assertive community treatment than with other types of intervention (3,5).

The evidence base for assertive community treatment is not without its limitations. For example, its effectiveness as a jail diversion program has not been clearly established, despite increasing interest in its use for this purpose (6). There is also widespread speculation that it may be less effective than more conventional treatments for individuals with personality disorders, although little hard evidence exists to either support or refute this idea (18). Also, its effectiveness for individuals from different ethnic groups has not been empirically established. Despite these limitations, assertive community treatment has many proven benefits, as noted above.

In many cases, assertive community treatment is not available to individuals who might benefit from this type of intervention (19). The purpose of this article is to familiarize mental health care providers with the principles of the assertive community treatment model and issues pertaining to its implementation. The article is a prelude to the detailed guidelines and strategies that are being developed as an implementation "toolkit" in the Evidence-Based Practices Project, an initiative funded by the Robert Wood Johnson Foundation and the Substance Abuse and Mental Health Services Administration (SAMHSA).

Principles of assertive community treatment

The practice of assertive community treatment originated almost 30 years ago when a group of mental health professionals at the Mendota Mental Health Institute in Wisconsin realized that many individuals with a severe mental illness were being discharged from inpatient care in stable condition, only to return after a relatively short time. Rather than accept the inevitability of repeated hospitalizations, these professionals looked at how mental health services were being delivered and tried to determine what could be done to help persons with mental illness live more stable lives in the community (20–23).

They designed a service delivery model in which a team of professionals assumes direct responsibility for providing the specific mix of services needed by a consumer, for as long as they are needed. The team ensures that services are available 24 hours a day, seven days a week. Rather than teaching skills or providing services in clinical settings and expecting them to be generalized to "real-life" situations, services are provided in vivo—that is, in the settings and context in which problems arise and support or skills are needed.

Team members collaborate to integrate the various interventions, and each consumer's response is carefully monitored so that interventions can be adjusted quickly to meet changing needs. Services are not limited to a predetermined set of interventions—they include any that are needed to support the consumer's optimal integration into the community (24). Rather than brokering services, the team itself is the service delivery vehicle in the model. Table 1 lists services provided by team members (25).

An assertive community treatment team consists of about ten to 12 staff members from the fields of psychiatry, nursing, and social work and professionals with other types of expertise, such as substance abuse treatment and vocational rehabilitation. Although the number of members may vary, the operating principle of the team is that it must be large enough to include representatives from the required disciplines and to provide coverage seven days a week, yet small enough so that each member is familiar with all the consumers served by the team. A staff-to-consumer ratio of one to ten is recommended, although teams that serve populations that have particularly intensive needs may find that a lower ratio is necessary initially. As the consumer population stabilizes, a higher ratio can be tolerated. A lower ratio may be appropriate in rural areas where considerable distances must be covered (22).

Team members are cross-trained in each other's areas of expertise to the maximum extent feasible, and they are readily available to assist and consult with each other. This team approach is facilitated by a daily review

Table 1

Services provided by assertive community treatment team members

Rehabilitative approach to daily living skills
  Grocery shopping and cooking
  Purchase and care of clothing
  Use of transportation
  Help with social and family relationships
Family involvement
  Crisis management
  Counseling and psychoeducation
    with family and extended family
  Coordination with family service
    agencies
Work opportunities
  Help to find volunteer and vocational
    opportunities
  Provide liaison with and educate
    employers
  Serve as job coach for consumers
Entitlements
  Assist with documentation
  Accompany consumers to entitlement
    offices
  Manage food stamps
  Assist with redetermination of benefits
Health promotion
  Provide preventive health education
  Conduct medical screening
  Schedule maintenance visits
  Provide liaison for acute medical care
  Provide reproductive counseling and
    sex education
Medication support
  Order medications from pharmacy
  Deliver medications to consumers
  Provide education about medication
  Monitor medication compliance and
    side effects
Housing assistance
  Find suitable shelter
  Secure leases and pay rent
  Purchase and repair household items
  Develop relationships with landlords
  Improve housekeeping skills
Financial management
  Plan budget
  Troubleshoot financial problems (for
    example, disability payments)
  Assist with bills
  Increase independence in money
    management
Counseling
  Use problem-oriented approach
  Integrate counseling into continuous
    work
  Ensure that goals are addressed by all
    team members
  Promote communication skills development
  Provide counseling as part of comprehensive rehabilitative approach

of each consumer's status and joint planning of the team members' daily activities (26).

Although this model of assertive

Table 2

Ten principles of assertive community treatment

Services are targeted to a specified group of individuals with severe mental illness.
Rather than brokering services, treatment, support, and rehabilitation services are
    provided directly by the assertive community treatment team.
Team members share responsibility for the individuals served by the team.
The staff-to-consumer ratio is small (approximately 1 to 10).
The range of treatment and services is comprehensive and flexible.
Interventions are carried out at the locations where problems occur and support is
    needed rather than in hospital or clinic settings.
There is no arbitrary time limit on receiving services.
Treatment and support services are individualized.
Services are available on a 24-hour basis.
The team is assertive in engaging individuals in treatment and monitoring their progress.

community treatment has been enhanced and modified to meet local needs or target specific clinical populations, its basic principles, which are summarized in Table 2, remain constant.

Variations on a theme

Assertive community treatment programs—with adaptations and enhancements—have been implemented in 35 states and in Canada, England, Sweden, and Australia (3,6,27). Programs operate in both urban and rural settings (8,27–32). Some emphasize outreach to homeless persons (33,34) or target veterans with severe mental illness (15,16,35). Others focus on co-occurring substance use disorders (10,17,36) or employment (21,37). Programs also differ in the extent to which they focus on personal growth or on basic survival (38). Some include consumers and family members as active members of the treatment teams (29,34).

Some program planners have questioned whether certain structural characteristics of assertive community treatment, such as the lack of a time limit on services, the team approach, and the provision of 24-hour crisis services, are overly expensive (39), and mental health authorities in some states have modified the model in terms of scope, eligibility, and programmatic features (6).

At the same time, several national organizations have promulgated standards to promote consistency among assertive community treatment programs. These standards differ from organization to organization. For instance, the standards developed by the National Alliance for the Mentally Ill (26) specify that programs be directly responsible for providing services to consumers 24 hours a day and for an unlimited time.

The standards promulgated by the Commission on Accreditation of Rehabilitation Facilities (40) allow for teams to arrange crisis coverage through other crisis intervention services. A recent directive from the VA (41) specifies that veterans may be shifted to less intensive care if explicit criteria for readiness are met after one year of assertive community treatment. Recommendations for staff-to-consumer ratios also vary among the different sets of standards.

The structural and operational elements addressed in the standards have potential fiscal consequences (6). For instance, it may be less costly for mental health systems to shift individuals to less intensive services than to provide assertive community treatment for a lifetime. Also, staffing an assertive community treatment team to provide 24-hour coverage rather than having consumers use existing crisis services on evenings and weekends will affect costs, as will variations in staff-to-consumer ratios.

Mental health systems will no doubt feel pressure to structure their programs in ways that minimize costs. However, current research does not provide detailed guidance for many of the decisions that program planners must make about the specifics of program structure. Program planners will want to keep in mind that the cost-effectiveness of assertive community treatment within a particular mental health system will depend not only on how the program is structured but also on the characteristics of the individuals targeted to receive treatment and the overall availability of mental health services in the community where a team operates.

There is some evidence that assertive community treatment is most cost-effective for individuals who have a history of high service use (15). Because hospital-based care is more expensive than community-based care, systems that target these individuals may realize greater cost savings. In communities where access to mental health services is limited, an assertive community treatment program may result in better access and, consequently, more effective treatment, but with higher service use and associated costs (8).

Critical program components

Given the variations among assertive community treatment programs in research studies and in actual practice, it would be helpful to program planners to know which core components are critical for effectiveness and which can be altered to fit local needs without affecting outcomes. Some specific program elements, such as a substance abuse treatment component and a supported employment component, have been linked to some specific favorable outcomes (9,37).

Most research, however, has focused on an aggregate of program elements, such as those described in the Dartmouth Assertive Community Treatment Fidelity Scale (DACTS) (42). The DACTS components, which are listed in Table 3, were compiled on the basis of an examination of the literature, expert consensus, and previous research on critical components of assertive community treatment (42–44). Some components codify basic characteristics of good clinical practice—for example, continuity of staff—rather than principles that differentiate assertive community treatment from other models—for example, in vivo services (Schaedle R, McGrew JH, Bond GR, unpublished data, 2000).

The results of research on assertive community treatment indicate that

Table 3

Indicators of high fidelity in an assertive community treatment program

Program component	Standard
Structure and human resources	
Small caseload	Ten or fewer consumers per clinician
Shared caseload	Provider group functions as a team rather than as individual practitioners
	Clinicians know and work with all consumers
	Ninety percent or more of consumers have contact with more than one staff member in one week
Program meeting	Program staff meet frequently to plan and review services for each consumer
	At least four program meetings per week, with each consumer reviewed during each meeting, if only briefly
Practicing team leader	Supervisor of frontline clinicians provides direct services at least 50 percent of the time
Continuity of staff	Program maintains same staffing over time, as evidenced by less than 20 percent turnover in two years
Staff capacity	Program operated at 95 percent or more of full staffing in the past 12 months
Psychiatrist on staff	At least one full-time psychiatrist is assigned directly to a program with 100 consumers
Nurse on staff	Two or more full-time nurses for a program with 100 consumers
Substance abuse specialist on staff	Two or more full-time employees with one year of substance abuse training or supervised substance abuse experience
Vocational specialist on staff	Two or more full-time employees with one year of vocational rehabilitation training or supervised vocational rehabilitation experience
Program size	Program is of sufficient absolute size to consistently provide the necessary staffing diversity and coverage (at least ten full-time employees)
Organizational boundaries	
Explicit admission criteria	Program has a clearly identified mission to serve a particular population and has and uses measurable and operationally defined criteria to screen out inappropriate referrals
	Program actively recruits a defined population, and all cases meet explicit admission criteria
Intake rate	Program takes consumers in at a low rate to maintain a stable service environment (highest monthly intake rate in the past six months was no greater than six consumers per month)
Full responsibility for treatment services	In addition to case management and psychiatric services, program directly provides counseling or psychotherapy, housing support, substance abuse treatment, employment, and rehabilitative services
Responsibility for crisis services	Program provides 24-hour coverage
Responsibility for hospital admissions	Ninety-five percent or more of admissions are initiated through the program
Responsibility for discharge planning	Ninety-five percent or more of discharges are planned jointly with the program
No time limit on services	Program never closes cases; it remains the point of contact for all consumers, as needed
Nature of services	
In vivo services	Program works to monitor status and develop community living skills in vivo rather than in the office; 80 percent of total service time is spent in the community
No-dropout policy	Program engages and retains consumers at a mutually satisfactory level; 95 percent or more of a caseload is retained over a 12-month period
Assertive engagement measures	Program demonstrates consistently well-thought-out strategies and uses street outreach and legal mechanisms whenever appropriate
Intensity of services	Large total amount of service time, as needed (on average, two hours or more per week per consumer)
Frequency of contact	Large number of service contacts, as needed (on average, four or more contacts per week per consumer)
Work with support system	With or without the consumer present, program provides support and skills for consumer's support network, including family, landlords, employers, and others (four or more contacts per month per consumer with support system in the community)
Individualized substance abuse treatment	One or more members of the program provide direct treatment and substance abuse treatment for consumers with substance use disorders
	Consumers with substance use disorders spend 24 minutes or more per week in substance abuse treatment
Dual disorder treatment groups	Program uses group modalities as a treatment strategy for people with substance use disorders
	Fifty percent or more of consumers with substance use disorders attend at least one substance abuse treatment group meeting per month
Dual disorders model	Program uses a stagewise treatment model that is nonconfrontational, follows behavioral principles, considers interactions of mental illness and substance abuse, and has gradual expectations of abstinence
	Program is fully based on dual disorders treatment principles, with treatment provided by program staff
Role of consumers on treatment team	Consumers are involved as members of the team, providing direct services
	Consumers are employed as clinicians (for example, case managers), with full professional status

programs that adhere overall to the DACTS components are more effective than programs with lower adherence in reducing hospital use (42), reducing costs (11), improving substance abuse outcomes for individuals with dual diagnoses (45,46), and improving functioning and consumers' quality of life (31,45). It should be noted that these studies compared assertive community treatment with standard care at the program level; the various specific structural components of assertive community treatment have not been systematically varied to determine their relative effects on outcomes.

The Lewin Group, a health services research firm under contract with the Health Care Finance Administration and SAMHSA, attempted to discern which of the various principles, structural elements, and organizational factors described in assertive community treatment standards and fidelity measures are most essential for successful outcomes (6). According to descriptions of programs in the literature, the characteristics most commonly reported in studies in which assertive community treatment produced better results than alternative treatments were found to be a team approach, in vivo services, assertive engagement, a small caseload, and explicit admission criteria. Although these findings suggest the importance of including these components in an assertive community treatment program, it should be noted that the study included only programs that adhered closely to the model and thus did not have the variability needed to determine the differential effects of any specific component on outcomes.

Other issues related to implementation

To our knowledge, no model for implementing an assertive community treatment program has been empirically tested. However, the principles and approaches found in research on changing health care practices should apply to this type of program. This research shows that, in general, successful implementation of new practices requires a leadership capable of initiating innovation, adequate financing, administrative rules and regulations that support the new practice, practitioners who have the skills necessary to carry out the new practice, and a means of providing feedback on the practice (2).

Because there has been no research specifically on methods for implementing assertive community treatment programs, the sources for the following discussion are observations of factors that hindered faithful replication of the assertive community treatment model in research studies; published manuals on implementing assertive community treatment, with contributions by the model's originators (22,26); telephone interviews with individuals experienced in implementing these types of programs; experiences in disseminating assertive community treatment programs within the VA; focus groups conducted by the Lewin Group with state mental health and Medicaid administrators; and numerous focus groups of consumers who have participated in assertive community treatment programs.

Implementation issues and strategies are presented for four key groups—mental health service system administrators, assertive community treatment program directors and team members (discussed together), and consumers.

Issues for mental health system administrators

Mental health system administrators are critical to the successful implementation of assertive community treatment programs. They provide the vision, set the goals, and ensure the instrumental support needed for the adoption of the model in routine practice. In this section, we address three issues that confront mental health system administrators: funding, ensuring adherence to the model, and planning the implementation of multiple programs.

Funding. Historically, funding for mental health services has been devoted primarily to the support of hospital-based and office-based care. One challenge in implementing assertive community treatment is that traditional funding streams may not cover the breadth of services provided for under the model. The primary source of funding for assertive community treatment is typically reimbursement through Medicaid under the rehabilitative services or targeted case management categories. In the VA, funding has been provided through special regional and national initiatives (47,48).

Reimbursement under Medicaid, when limited to the parameters of the rehabilitative services or targeted case management categories, does not always cover all the services provided by an assertive community treatment team, such as failed attempts to contact an individual. Some states have augmented Medicaid funding by blending Medicaid reimbursement with funds from other sources, such as revenues for substance abuse treatment or housing. Because each funding stream has separate requirements that are often contradictory, blended funding can be cumbersome; however, it does offer a potential solution to the limitations of Medicaid funding (6).

New Hampshire and Rhode Island have addressed the limitations of Medicaid by revising their state plans to cover the services provided by assertive community treatment teams. States may find that consultation with a Medicaid expert is helpful in developing financial constructs to cover assertive community treatment services.

Ensuring adherence to the model. It is not uncommon for health care programs to depart from the model they seek to replicate. Variations may be intentional, such as those introduced in response to local conditions (6,38). Variations may also occur when shortages of resources place pressure on administrators to make trade-offs between program effectiveness and program costs. Finally, unintended variations may occur, such as when the model is not clearly understood, when the training provided is inadequate, or when staff members regress to previous, more familiar practices (38).

A number of safeguards can be instituted by system administrators to prevent unintended variations. First, mental health systems can include standards for assertive community treatment programs in state plans (22,49,50). However, a survey of states that have assertive community treatment initiatives found that the standards enacted by individual states often failed to address many elements included in the DACTS or they lacked specificity (50). Since the survey was conducted, SAMHSA has supported the development of national standards for assertive community treatment programs that can serve as a model for state standards (26).

Implementing the multilevel changes needed to disseminate a program model such as assertive community treatment throughout a state system may take three to five years—a period that exceeds the tenure of most state mental health directors (49). A steering committee that is contractually mandated by the state mental health authority and that serves in an oversight capacity can help to ensure that initiatives are sustained as administrations change over time. Advisory groups with multiple stakeholders can play a similar role at the team or agency level. The advisory group can serve as a liaison between the community and the treatment team and other bodies within the provider agency. Such groups are currently used in programs in Tennessee, Montana, Florida, and Oklahoma.

Advisory groups should include individuals who are knowledgeable about severe mental illness and the challenges that people with mental illness face in living in the community; consumers of mental health services and their relatives; and community stakeholders who have an interest in the success of the assertive community treatment team, such as representatives of homeless services, the criminal justice system, consumer peer support organizations, and community colleges, as well as landlords and employers.

Well-delineated training, supervision, and consultation can help to ensure that the model is understood initially by the practitioners who will carry out the program; however, ongoing monitoring of program fidelity is also important for continued efficiency and effectiveness (47,48,50). The DACTS can be used either by persons within the mental health system or by external experts to measure a program's adherence to the model

(42). This instrument is useful for ensuring appropriate initial implementation as well as maintenance of fidelity over time (47,48,51).

Multiple programs. Experience suggests that states implementing multiple programs will want to consider the pace at which new teams are started (38). Some states, such as New Jersey and Pennsylvania, have successfully launched multiple programs simultaneously. The concurrent development of teams allows for shared training, which can increase the connections between newly forming teams, enhance practitioners' understanding of the model, help counteract the isolation of individual teams, and encourage mutual problem solving (38). On the other hand, implementing teams sequentially allows systems to use teams that were trained early in the implementation effort to mentor and monitor subsequent teams. The VA has used this approach to implement 50 teams over the past decade (47,51).

Another strategy to facilitate the implementation of multiple programs is to appoint a clinical coordinator who is experienced in assertive community treatment and who has frequent, ongoing contact with each new program to assist with and assess implementation. This individual provides ongoing formal and informal training and plays an important role in the early detection of potential problems (52).

Issues for program directors and team members

There is evidence in the literature—and unanimity among the experts we interviewed—that successful replication of assertive community treatment programs is facilitated when program directors have a clear concept of the model's goals and treatment principles (42). Program directors who are committed to the model are better able to hold the staff accountable for fidelity to the model and to provide the leadership and instrumental support needed to ensure its successful adoption by staff. Visits by program directors and team members to existing programs with proven fidelity and ongoing mentoring by someone experienced with the model

are highly recommended (22,31).

Policies and procedures. Existing agency policies may not cover all activities of an assertive community treatment team. For example, team members routinely transport individuals, an activity that may not be addressed in the policy and procedures of office-based programs. Some programs address this issue by reimbursing team members for the cost of insurance and operating expenses for their personal vehicles. Other programs elect to have team members use agency vehicles.

Another issue that requires forethought is how medication delivery will be accomplished. Team members, both medical and nonmedical, may at times deliver medications to individuals in the community. Because nonmedical personnel cannot dispense medications, some programs establish procedures whereby consumers set up their own medications in "organizers" so that nonmedical personnel can make deliveries.

Yet another issue that administrators and staff may be concerned about is the safety of team members when they are out in the community. Teams often find that cell phones provide reassurance and also facilitate nonemergency communication.

More detailed discussions of these issues can be found in other publications (22,26). Actual model policies are available in the PACT start-up manual (26).

Selecting and retaining team members. Methods for providing assertive community treatment may differ considerably from those that professional staff have been exposed to previously. For example, members of an assertive community treatment team work interdependently, and the majority of their time is spent in community settings. Pragmatism, street smarts, initiative, and the ability to work with a group are particularly desirable characteristics for team members (22). Competitive salaries are important in attracting and retaining competent individuals (6,26,38).

As noted, mental health consumers hold positions on some assertive community treatment teams (29,34). Personal experience with mental illness is thought to afford these individuals a unique perspective on the mental health system. At the same time, concerns have been expressed that consumers may be more vulnerable than others to the stress associated with providing mental health services and the difficulties of maintaining boundaries and that they may face stigmatization by other professionals (53,54). There are no data to suggest that consumers should be restricted from filling any position on a team for which they might be qualified. When consumers fill the role of peer specialist rather than other professional roles, their services may not be covered by third-party reimbursement (55), and programs will need to identify other revenues to fund these positions (6).

Training. Implementing assertive community treatment involves changing the type of work staff members may be used to as well as the manner in which they work. Working in community-based care also casts a different light on a staff member's cultural competency and professional boundaries.

Consultants who have been involved in implementing successful teams suggest that members of a new team shadow an experienced team, that they receive several full days of didactic training before program start-up, and that they take part in intermittent booster training sessions. This training sequence can be supplemented with videos, manuals, and workbooks, some of which are currently under development and will take the form of an implementation toolkit that will be tested in the field.

As newly forming teams encounter the pressures of a growing caseload, it is tempting to resort to the more traditional individual case management practice. Continuous on-site and telephone supervision is important in helping new teams maintain a shared-caseload approach (21,22,26,56–60).

Organizational integration of the team. The relationship between the assertive community treatment team and the larger system of care is also important. At one extreme, a team can be too detached from the larger system, either because it is physically isolated or because other programs view the team as special-ized and the team's activities as unrelated to their own daily activities.

A degree of detachment can help to ensure that the team takes primary responsibility for providing a full range of services rather than relying on programs in the larger service delivery system. On the other hand, if a team is too detached, it may have difficulty developing channels of formal and informal communication with professionals in the larger service system. If the team is too autonomous or appears aloof, team members will find it difficult to successfully broker services for consumers when they are needed (31,59).

At the other extreme, problems can arise when a team cannot make independent decisions consistent with program principles because of expectations imposed on it by the larger organization. For instance, in a case in which assertive community treatment was attempted with individuals who had severe mental illness and mental retardation and who were living in a group home, the policies and practices of the mental retardation program were imposed on the assertive community treatment team. The team found it difficult to adhere to the practices of the mental retardation program and at the same time put the core principles of the assertive community treatment model into practice (61).

It is also sometimes difficult for assertive community treatment to emerge as an autonomous program, in part because other programs operating within a conceptual framework of compartmentalized service delivery may find it difficult to understand the assertive community treatment model (38). When teams lack autonomy, it is difficult to respond to consumers' changing needs in a manner consistent with the principles of the model (31,61).

Adequate channels of communication and respect for the autonomy of the team can be facilitated when other programs operating within the system and in the community have a clear idea of the goals and methods of the assertive community treatment program. Systemwide training in the principles of the model can help in this regard.

Issues for consumers

Studies have found that individuals who receive assertive community treatment report greater general satisfaction with their care than those who receive other services (5). However, some consumer groups strongly oppose the widespread dissemination of assertive community treatment. They believe that it is a mechanism for exerting social control over individuals who have a mental illness, particularly through the use of medications; that it can be coercive; that it is paternalistic; and that it may foster dependency (62–64).

A recent study of strategies used by assertive community treatment teams to pressure consumers to change behaviors or to stay in treatment shows that more coercive interventions, such as committing individuals to a hospital against their will, were used with less that 10 percent of consumers. More coercive interventions were used most often when consumers had recent substance abuse problems, a history of arrest, an extensive history of hospitalization, or more severe symptoms (65). An earlier study of consumers who were receiving assertive community treatment found that about one of every ten believed that the treatment was too intrusive or confining or that it fostered dependency (66).

It may not be possible to satisfy the concerns of consumer groups that object on principle to the assertive community treatment model, but it is important to acknowledge that this practice, like any other, has some potential to be used in a coercive manner. The issue of coercion may be of particular concern when this model is used in conjunction with outpatient commitment or in forensic settings, where staff must balance their clinical role with their legal responsibilities (6,55).

The idea that assertive community treatment is paternalistic may stem from the assumption that once individuals are deemed to be appropriate candidates for this service, they will require the same level of service for life. This assumption is called into question by studies suggesting that it is possible to transfer stabilized individuals to less intensive services with no adverse consequences (16, 67,68).

Consumers' dissatisfaction with the treatments offered by the mental health system has a basis in their own experiences. Mental health providers can become more aware of consumers' concerns about assertive community treatment when consumers take an active part in state and local advisory groups and serve as team members. Also, research on consumers' perspectives on assertive community treatment, which has been limited largely to studies of consumer satisfaction, needs to be expanded (62).

Differing viewpoints about assertive community treatment—as well as about other forms of mental health treatment—are to be expected, and it is important that providers be aware of them. Furthermore, individuals who do not want to use assertive community treatment services should be able to select from alternative services along a continuum of care, even when such services do not have as strong an evidence base as assertive community treatment.

Conclusions
Since the inception of assertive community treatment nearly 30 years ago, research has repeatedly demonstrated that it reduces hospitalization, increases housing stability, and improves the quality of life for those individuals with severe mental illness who experience the most intractable symptoms and experience the greatest impairment as a result of mental illness. This model of delivering integrated, community-based treatment, support, and rehabilitation services has been adapted to a variety of settings, circumstances, and populations.

Although research shows that greater adherence to a group of core principles produces better outcomes, the relationship between specific structural aspects of assertive community treatment programs and outcomes is not always clear. When this model is being implemented, thoughtful consideration should be given to research on assertive community treatment programs and local conditions. Issues that should be considered include adequate funding, monitoring of fi-

delity, adaptation of policies and procedures to accommodate the model, and adequate training of professional staff. Tools that provide practical information on how to address issues related to implementing the assertive community treatment model will be available in the near future. ◆

Acknowledgments
This article was written in conjunction with the Evidence-Based Practices Project sponsored by the Center for Mental Health Services and the Robert Wood Johnson Foundation. It is supported by grant 280-00-8049 from the Substance Abuse and Mental Health Services Administration. The authors thank Paul Gorman, M.Ed., and Gary R. Bond, Ph.D., for their comments and suggestions.

References
1. Mental Health: A Report of the Surgeon General. Rockville, Md, Substance Abuse and Mental Health Services Administration, Center for Mental Health Services, 1999
2. Torrey WC, Drake RE, Dixon L, et al: Implementing evidence-based practices for persons with severe mental illnesses. Psychiatric Services 52:45–55, 2001
3. Burns BJ, Santos AB: Assertive community treatment: an update of randomized trials. Psychiatric Services 46:669–675, 1995
4. Bedell JR, Cohen NL, Sullivan A: Case management: the current best practices and the next generation of innovation. Community Mental Health Journal 36:179–194, 2000
5. Bond GR, Drake RE, Mueser KT, et al: Assertive community treatment for people with severe mental illness: critical ingredients and impact on consumers. Disease Management and Health Outcomes 9:141–159, 2001
6. Assertive Community Treatment Literature Review. Falls Church, Va, Lewin Group, 2000
7. Taube CA, Morlock L, Burns BJ, et al: New Directions in Research on Community Treatment. Hospital and Community Psychiatry 41:642–647, 1990
8. Mueser K, Bond GR, Drake RE, et al: Models of community care for severe mental illness: a review of research on case management. Schizophrenia Bulletin 24:37–74, 1998
9. Drake RE, McHugo G, Clark R, et al: Assertive community treatment for patients with co-occurring severe mental illness and substance use disorder: a clinical trial. American Journal of Orthopsychiatry 68:201–213, 1998
10. Teague GB, Drake RE, Ackerson T: Evaluating use of continuous treatment teams for persons with mental illness and substance abuse. Psychiatric Services 46:689–695, 1995

11. Latimer E: Economic impacts of assertive community treatment: a review of the literature. Canadian Journal of Psychiatry 44:443–454, 1999
12. Wolff LI, Barry KL, Dien GV, et al: Estimated societal costs of assertive community mental health care. Psychiatric Services 46:898–906, 1995
13. Essock S, Frisman L, Kontos N: Cost-effectiveness of assertive community treatment teams. American Journal of Orthopsychiatry 68:179–190, 1998
14. Lehman A, Dixon L, Hoch J, et al: Cost-effectiveness of assertive community treatment for homeless persons with severe mental illness. British Journal of Psychiatry 174:346–352, 1999
15. Rosenheck RA, Neale M, Leaf P, et al: Multisite experimental cost study of intensive psychiatric community care. Schizophrenia Bulletin 21:129–140, 1995
16. Rosenheck RA, Neale M: Intersite variation in the impact of intensive psychiatric community care on hospital use. American Journal of Orthopsychiatry 68:191–200, 1998
17. Clark RE, Teague GB, Ricketts SD, et al: Cost-effectiveness of assertive community treatment versus standard case management for persons with co-occurring severe mental illness and substance use disorders. Health Services Research 33:1285–1308, 1998
18. Weisbrod BA: A guide to cost-benefit analysis, as seen through a controlled experiment in treating the mentally ill. Journal of Health Politics, Policy, and Law 7:808–847, 1983
19. Lehman AF, Steinwachs DM: Survey co-investigators of the PORT project: Translating research into practice: the Schizophrenia Patient Outcomes Research Team (PORT) treatment recommendations. Schizophrenia Bulletin 24:1–10, 1998
20. Marx AJ, Test MA, Stein LI: Extrahospital management of severe mental illness: feasibility and effects of social functioning. Archives of General Psychiatry 29:505–511, 1973
21. Stein LI: Innovating Against the Current. Madison, Mental Health Research Center, University of Wisconsin, 1992
22. Stein LI, Santos AB: Assertive Community Treatment of Persons With Severe Mental Illness. New York, Norton, 1998
23. Test MA: Training in community living, in Handbook of Psychiatric Rehabilitation. Edited by Liberman RP. New York, Macmillan, 1992
24. Stein LI, Test MA: Alternative to mental hospital treatment: I. conceptual model, treatment program, and clinical evaluation. Archives of General Psychiatry 37:400–405, 1980
25. Burns BJ, Swartz MS: Hospital Without Walls: Videotape Study Guide. Durham, NC, Division of Social and Community Psychiatry, Department of Psychiatry, Duke University Medical Center, 1994
26. Allness DJ, Knoedler WH: The PACT

Model of Community-Based Treatment for Persons With Severe and Persistent Mental Illnesses: A Manual for PACT Start-Up. Arlington, Va, National Alliance for the Mentally Ill, 1999

27. Deci PA, Santos AB, Hiott DW, et al: Dissemination of assertive community treatment programs. Psychiatric Services 46:676–678, 1995

28. Rapp C: The active ingredients of effective case management: a research synthesis. Community Mental Health Journal 34:363–380, 1998

29. Dixon LB, Stewart B, Krauss N, et al: The participation of families of homeless persons with severe mental illness in an outreach intervention. Community Mental Health Journal 34:251–259, 1998

30. Lehman A, Dixon L, Kernan E, et al: A randomized trial of assertive community treatment for homeless persons with severe mental illness. Archives of General Psychiatry 54:1038–1043, 1997

31. McDonel EC, Bond GR, Salyers M, et al: Implementing assertive community treatment programs in rural settings. Administration and Policy in Mental Health 25:153–173, 1997

32. Santos AB, Deci PA, Dias JK, et al: Providing assertive community treatment for severely mentally ill patients in a rural area. Hospital and Community Psychiatry 44:34–39, 1993

33. Tsemberis S, Eisenberg RF: Pathways to housing: supported housing for street-dwelling homeless individuals with psychiatric disabilities. Psychiatric Services 51:487–505, 2000

34. Morse GA, Caslyn RJ, Allen G, et al: Experimental comparison of the effects of three treatment programs for homeless mentally ill people. Hospital and Community Psychiatry 43:1005–1009, 1992

35. Rosenheck RA, Neale M: Cost-effectiveness of intensive psychiatric community care for high users of inpatient services. Archives of General Psychiatry 55:459–466,1998

36. Bond GR, McDonel EC, Miller LD, et al: Assertive community treatment and reference groups: an evaluation of their effectiveness for young adults with serious mental illness and substance abuse problems. Psychosocial Rehabilitation Journal 15:31–43, 1991

37. Drake RE, McHugo GJ, Becker DR, et al: The New Hampshire study of supported employment for people with severe mental illness. Journal of Consulting and Clinical Psychology 64:391–399, 1996

38. Bond G: Variations in an assertive outreach model. New Directions for Mental Health Services 52:65–80, 1991

39. McGrew JH, Bond GR: The association between program characteristics and service delivery in assertive community treatment. Administration and Policy in Mental Health 25:175–189, 1997

40. Assertive community treatment, in CARF 2000 Behavioral Health Standards Manual. Tucson, Ariz, Commission on Accreditation of Rehabilitation Facilities, 2000

41. VHA Mental Health Intensive Case Management (MHICM): VHA Directive 2000-034. Washington, DC, Veterans Health Administration, Department of Veterans Affairs, 2000

42. Teague GB, Bond GR, Drake RE: Program fidelity in assertive community treatment: development and use of a measure. American Journal of Orthopsychiatry 68:216–232, 1998

43. McGrew J, Bond GR: Critical ingredients of assertive community treatment: judgments of the experts. Journal of Mental Health Administration 22:113–125,1995

44. McGrew JH, Bond GR, Dietzen L, et al: Measuring the fidelity of implementation of a mental health program model. Journal of Consulting and Clinical Psychology 62:113–125, 1994

45. McHugo GJ, Drake RE, Teague GB: Fidelity to assertive community treatment and consumer outcomes in the New Hampshire dual disorders study. Psychiatric Services 50:818–824, 1999

46. Fekete DM, Bond GR, McDonel EC, et al: Rural intensive case management: a controlled study. Psychiatric Rehabilitation Journal 21:371–379, 1998

47. Rosenheck RA, Neale M, Baldino R, et al: Intensive Psychiatric Community Care: A New Approach to Care for Veterans With Serious Mental Illness in the Department of Veterans Affairs. West Haven, Conn, Northeast Program Evaluation Center, 1997

48. Rosenheck RA, Neale M: Development, implementation, and monitoring of intensive psychiatric community care in the Department of Veterans Affairs, in Achieving Quality in Psychiatric and Substance Abuse Practice: Concepts and Case Reports. Edited by Dickey B, Sederer L. Washington, DC, American Psychiatric Press, in press

49. Santos AB, Henggler SW, Burns BJ, et al: Research on field-based services: models for reform in the delivery of mental health care to populations with complex clinical problems. American Journal of Psychiatry 152:1111–1123, 1995

50. Meisler N: Assertive community treatment initiatives: results from a survey of selected state mental health authorities. Community Support Network News 11:3–5, 1997

51. Neale M, Rosenheck RA, Baldino R, et al: Intensive Psychiatric Community Care (IPCC), in the Department of Veterans Affairs Third National Performance Monitoring Report FY 1999. West Haven, Conn, Northeast Program Evaluation Center, VA Connecticut Healthcare System, Department of Veterans Affairs, 2000

52. McGrew JH, Bond GR, Dietzen LL, et al: A multisite study of client outcomes in assertive community treatment. Psychiatric Services 4:696–701, 1995

53. Paulson R, Herinckx H, Demmler J, et al: Comparing practice patterns of consumer and non-consumer mental health service providers. Community Mental Health Journal 35:251–269, 1999

54. Felton CJ, Stastny P, Shern DL, et al: Consumers as peer specialists on intensive case management teams: impact on clients. Psychiatric Services 46:1037–1044, 1995

55. Solomon P, Draine J: One-year outcomes of a randomized trial of case management with seriously mentally ill clients leaving jail. Evaluation Review 19: 256–274, 1995

56. Rutkowski P, Plum T, McCarthy D, et al: P/ACT dissemination and implementation from three states and the Department of Veterans Affairs. Community Support Network News 11:8–9, 1997

57. Cook JA, Horton-O'Connell T, Fitzgibbon G, et al: Training for state-funded providers of assertive community treatment. New Directions in Mental Health Services, 79:55–64, 1998

58. Hadley TR, Roland T, Vasko S, et al: Community treatment teams: an alternative to state hospital. Psychiatric Quarterly 68:77–90, 1997

59. Stein LI, Test MA: Retraining hospital staff for work in a community program in Wisconsin. Hospital and Community Psychiatry 27:266–268, 1976

60. Witheridge TF: The assertive community treatment worker: an emerging role and its implications for professional training. Hospital and Community Psychiatry 40:620–624, 1989

61. Meisler N, McKay CD, Gold PB, et al: Using principles of ACT to integrate community care for people with mental retardation and mental illness. Journal of Psychiatric Practice 6:77–83, 2000

62. Spindel P, Nugent J: The Trouble With PACT: Questioning the Increasing Use of Assertive Community Treatment Teams in Community Mental Health. Consumer Organization and Networking Technical Assistance Center, Charleston, WV. Available at http://www.contac.org/nec.htm

63. Fischer DB, Ahern L: Personal Assistance in Community Existence (PACE): an alternative to PACT. Ethical Human Sciences and Services 2:87–92, 2000

64. Estroff S: Making It Crazy: An Ethnographic Study of Psychiatric Clients in an American Community. Berkeley, University of California Press, 1981

65. Neale M, Rosenheck RA: Therapeutic limit setting in an assertive community treatment program. Psychiatric Services 51:499–505, 2000

66. McGrew JH, Wilson R, Bond GR: Client perspectives on critical ingredients of assertive community treatment. Psychiatric Rehabilitation Journal 19:13–21, 1996

67. Salyers MP, Masterton TW, Fekete DM, et al: Transferring clients from intensive case management: impact on client functioning. American Journal of Orthopsychiatry 68:233–245, 1998

68. Susser E, Valencia E, Conover S, et al: Preventing recurrent homelessness among mentally ill men: a "critical time" intervention after discharge from a shelter. American Journal of Public Health 87:256–262, 1997

Evidence-Based Practices for Services to Families of People With Psychiatric Disabilities

Lisa Dixon, M.D., M.P.H.
William R. McFarlane, M.D.
Harriet Lefley, Ph.D.
Alicia Lucksted, Ph.D.
Michael Cohen, M.A.
Ian Falloon, M.D.
Kim Mueser, Ph.D.
David Miklowitz, Ph.D.
Phyllis Solomon, Ph.D.
Diane Sondheimer, M.S., M.P.H.

Family psychoeducation is an evidence-based practice that has been shown to reduce relapse rates and facilitate recovery of persons who have mental illness. A core set of characteristics of effective family psychoeducation programs has been developed, including the provision of emotional support, education, resources during periods of crisis, and problem-solving skills. Unfortunately, the use of family psychoeducation in routine practice has been limited. Barriers at the level of the consumer and his or her family members, the clinician and the administrator, and the mental health authority reflect the existence of attitudinal, knowledge-based, practical, and systemic obstacles to implementation. Family psychoeducation dissemination efforts that have been successful to date have built consensus at all levels, including among consumers and their family members; have provided ample training, technical assistance, and supervision to clinical staff; and have maintained a long-term perspective.

Dr. Dixon and Dr. Lucksted are affiliated with the Center for Mental Health Services Research at the University of Maryland School of Medicine in Baltimore and with the Department of Veterans Affairs Capitol Health Care Network Mental Illness Research, Education, and Clinical Center, 701 West Pratt Street, Room 476, Baltimore, Maryland 21201 (e-mail, ldixon@umaryland.edu). Dr. McFarlane is affiliated with the Maine Medical Center in Portland. Dr. Lefley is with the University of Miami School of Medicine. Mr. Cohen is with the New Hampshire chapter of the National Alliance for the Mentally Ill in Concord. Dr. Falloon is with the University of Auckland in Auckland, New Zealand. Dr. Mueser is with Dartmouth Medical School in Hanover, New Hampshire. Dr. Miklowitz is with the University of Colorado. Dr. Solomon is with the University of Pennsylvania School of Social Work in Philadelphia. Ms. Sondheimer is with the Child, Adolescent, and Family Branch of the Center for Mental Health Services in Rockville, Maryland. This article was originally published in the July 2001 issue of Psychiatric Services.

Family members and other persons involved in the lives and care of adults who have serious mental illnesses often provide emotional support, case management, financial assistance, advocacy, and housing to their mentally ill loved ones. Although serving in this capacity can be rewarding, it imposes considerable burdens (1–4). Family members often have limited access to the resources and information they need (5–7). Research conducted over the past decade has shown that patients' outcomes improve when the needs of family members for information, clinical guidance, and support are met. This research supports the development of evidence-based practice guidelines for addressing the needs of family members.

Several models have evolved to address the needs of families of persons with mental illness: individual consultation and family psychoeducation conducted by a mental health professional (8,9), various forms of more traditional family therapy (10), and a range of professionally led short-term family education programs (11,12), sometimes referred to as therapeutic education. Also available are family-led information and support classes or groups, such as those provided by the National Alliance for the Mentally Ill (NAMI) (13,14). Family psychoeducation has a deep enough research and dissemination base to be considered an evidenced-based practice. However, the term "psychoeducation" can be misleading: family psychoeducation includes many therapeutic elements, often uses a consultative framework, and shares characteristics with other types of family interventions.

In general, evidence-based practices are clinical practices for which scientific evidence of improvement in consumer outcomes has been consistent (15). The scientific evidence of the highest standard is the randomized clinical trial. Often, several clinical trials are pooled by use of a technique such as meta-analysis to identify evidence-based practices. Quasi-experimental studies, and to a lesser extent open clinical trials, can also be used. However, the research evidence for an evidence-based practice must be consistent and sufficiently specific for the quality and outcome of the intervention to be assessed.

The purpose of this article, as part of a larger series on evidenced-based practices for persons with severe mental illnesses (15), is to describe family psychoeducation, the basis for its identification as an evidence-based practice, and barriers to its implementation. We also propose strategies for overcoming these barriers.

What is family psychoeducation?

A variety of family psychoeducation programs have been developed by mental health care professionals over the past two decades (8,9). These programs have been offered as part of an overall clinical treatment plan for individuals who have mental illness. They last nine months to five years, are usually diagnosis specific, and focus primarily on consumer outcomes, although the well-being of the family is an essential intermediate outcome. Family psychoeducation models differ in their format—for example, multiple-family, single-family, or mixed sessions—the duration of treatment, consumer participation, location—for example, clinic based, home, family practice,

or other community settings—and the degree of emphasis on didactic, cognitive-behavioral, and systemic techniques.

Although the existing models of family intervention appear to differ from one another, a strong consensus about the critical elements of family intervention emerged in 1999 under the encouragement of the leaders of the World Schizophrenia Fellowship (16).

Goals and principles for working with families

The main goals in working with the family of a person who has a mental illness are to achieve the best possible outcome for the patient through collaborative treatment and management and to alleviate the suffering of the family members by supporting them in their efforts to aid the recovery of their loved one.

Treatment models that have been supported by evidence of effectiveness have required clinicians to adhere to 15 principles in working with families of persons who have mental illness:

♦ Coordinate all elements of treatment and rehabilitation to ensure that everyone is working toward the same goals in a collaborative, supportive relationship.

♦ Pay attention to both the social and the clinical needs of the consumer.

♦ Provide optimum medication management.

♦ Listen to families' concerns and involve them as equal partners in the planning and delivery of treatment.

♦ Explore family members' expectations of the treatment program and expectations for the consumer.

♦ Assess the strengths and limitations of the family's ability to support the consumer.

♦ Help resolve family conflict by responding sensitively to emotional distress.

♦ Address feelings of loss.

♦ Provide relevant information for the consumer and his or her family at appropriate times.

♦ Provide an explicit crisis plan and professional response.

♦ Help improve communication among family members.

♦ Provide training for the family in

structured problem-solving techniques.

♦ Encourage family members to expand their social support networks—for example, to participate in family support organizations such as NAMI.

♦ Be flexible in meeting the needs of the family.

♦ Provide the family with easy access to another professional in the event that the current work with the family ceases.

Overview of the research

Studies have shown markedly higher reductions in relapse and rehospitalization rates among consumers whose families received psychoeducation than among those who received standard individual services (17–20), with differences ranging from 20 to 50 percent over two years. For programs of more than three months' duration, the reductions in relapse rates were at the higher end of this range. In addition, the well-being of family members improved (21), patients' participation in vocational rehabilitation increased (22), and the costs of care decreased (4,20,23,24).

As a result of this compelling evidence, the Schizophrenia Patient Outcomes Research Team (PORT) included family psychoeducation among its treatment recommendations. The PORT recommended that all families who have contact with a relative who has mental illness be offered a family psychosocial intervention that spans at least nine months and that includes education about mental illness, family support, crisis intervention, and problem ·solving (25). Other best-practice standards (26–28) have recommended that families participate in education and support programs. In addition, an expert panel that included clinicians from various disciplines as well as families, consumers, and researchers emphasized the importance of engaging family members in the treatment and rehabilitation of persons who are mentally ill (29,30).

Delivering the appropriate components of family psychoeducation for patients and their families appears to be an important determinant of outcomes for both consumers and their families. It has been demonstrated that programs do not reduce relapse rates if the information presented is not accompanied by skills training, ongoing guidance about management of mental illness, and emotional support for family members (31).

In addition, these interventions that present information in isolation tend to be brief: a meta-analysis of 16 studies found that family interventions of fewer than ten sessions had no substantial effects on the burden of family members (32). However, the number of sessions could not completely explain the differences in outcomes. The outcomes may have been influenced by the total duration of treatment rather than the number of sessions, or by the individual therapist's approach to dealing with the emotional reactions of patients and their families. The behaviors and disruptions associated with schizophrenia, in particular, may require more than education to ameliorate the burden on the family and enhance consumer outcomes.

Most studies have evaluated family psychoeducation for schizophrenia or schizoaffective disorder only. However, the results of several controlled studies support the benefits of both single- and multiple-family interventions for other psychiatric disorders, including bipolar disorder (33–38), major depression (39–41), obsessive-compulsive disorder (42), anorexia nervosa (43), and borderline personality disorder (44). Gonzalez and colleagues (45) have extended this research to deal with the secondary effects of chronic physical illness.

Family psychoeducation thus has a solid research base, and leaders in the field have reached consensus on the essential components and techniques of family psychoeducation. This form of treatment should continue to be recommended for use in routine practice. However, several important gaps remain in the knowledge required to make comprehensive evidence-based practice recommendations and to implement them with a wide variety of families.

First, although the members of the World Schizophrenia Fellowship and others have delineated the core components of a successful family intervention, the minimum ingredients

are still not clear. This gap was highlighted by a study of treatment strategies for schizophrenia, which found no significant difference in relapse rates between families who received a relatively intensive program—a simplified version of cognitive-behavioral family intervention plus a multiple family group—and those who received a less intensive psychoeducational, or supportive, multiple-family group program (46). However, both programs provided levels of support and education to families that far surpassed those provided by usual services. It will be necessary to conduct studies designed to identify the least intensive and smallest effective "dose" of family psychoeducation.

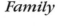

Family psychoeducation has a solid research base, and leaders in the field have reached consensus on its essential components and techniques.

Second, increasing the sophistication, variety, and scope of indicators that are used to measure "benefit" is essential. Commonly used benchmarks are subject to complicated intervening variables and need to be correlated with other results. For example, a greater number of hospitalizations for a mentally ill person during the year after family psychoeducation could be a positive sign if it indicates that a previously neglected consumer is getting care and that the family is getting better at identifying prodromal symptoms that indicate an impending relapse (4). The well-being and health of the family should be routinely measured as well.

A third knowledge gap involves the

relationship between family psychoeducation and other programs. Since the conception of family psychoeducation, other psychosocial programs have developed a substantial evidentiary base, including supported employment and assertive community treatment (47,48). For example, assertive community treatment combined with family psychoeducation has been associated with better noncompetitive employment outcomes than assertive community treatment alone (22). The combination of assertive community treatment, family psychoeducation, and supported employment has been associated with better competitive employment outcomes than conventional vocational rehabilitation, although the contributions of each component could not be assessed in that study (49). The opportunities for family psychoeducation to be combined with or compared with these new psychosocial models have not been fully explored.

Fourth, research is needed to refine the interventions so that they better address different types of families, different situations, and different time points throughout the course of illness. For example, there is some evidence that individualized consultation may be more beneficial than group psychoeducation for families who have existing sources of support or who already belong to a support group (50–52).

Fifth, although family psychoeducation has been tested in a wide range of national and global settings, there is still a need to assess modifications in content and outcome among particular U.S. subcultures and in other countries. In the United States the one study involving Latino families had mixed results (53,54). However, studies in China (55–57) as well as studies that are under way among Vietnamese refugees living in Australia have had results comparable to those of studies conducted in Caucasian populations.

Finally, what happens after a family has completed a psychoeducation program? Families of consumers with long-term problems and disability may need ongoing support and enhanced problem-solving skills to deal with the vicissitudes of illness. Lefley

(58) has described ad hoc psychoeducation in informal settings, such as an ongoing family support group conducted through a medical center. McFarlane (4,59) has used a usually open-ended multiple-family group structure. NAMI's Family-to-Family program is limited to 12 sessions of formal education but offers continuity in the NAMI support and educational group structure (14).

Barriers to implementation

Despite the gaps in the research, the extensive documentation of the basic benefits of family psychoeducation prompts the question of why this service is rarely offered. In general, low levels of contact between clinical staff and family members in public and community-based settings may preclude the more substantial educational or support interventions. Also, the availability of any intervention is limited by the availability of people to provide it and the training necessary to equip those people. The requisite clinicians, resources, time, and reimbursement have not been forthcoming. These deficits imply the existence of larger obstacles related to attitudes, knowledge, practicality, and systems.

Consumers and family members

Implementation of family psychoeducation may be hindered by realities in the lives of potential participants. Practical impediments such as transportation problems and competing demands for time and energy are common (50). If family members perceive that the training provided through family psychoeducation involves expectations of additional caregiving responsibilities, they may stay away (16). Sessions must be scheduled during periods when facilitators are available, but these times may not suit the clients and their families. Family members face significant burdens that may pose barriers to attending family psychoeducation sessions, even though attendance could lighten these burdens (60,61).

In addition, stigma is common—family members may not want to be identified with psychiatric facilities. They may feel uncomfortable revealing that there is psychiatric illness in their family and airing their problems in a public setting. They may have had negative experiences in the past and be hesitant to expose themselves to the possibility of further negative experiences. Most people have not had access to information about the value of family psychoeducation and so may not appreciate the potential utility of these programs (16). They may believe that nothing will help. Consumers may have similar apprehensions and may worry about losing the confidential relationship with their treatment teams or about losing autonomy.

Clinicians and program administrators

The lack of availability of family psychoeducation may reflect an underappreciation on the part of mental health care providers of the utility and importance of this treatment approach (16,18,31,50). Providers may choose medication over psychosocial interventions, and family involvement may seem superfluous. In addition, some providers may still adhere to theories that blame family dynamics for schizophrenia. Bergmark (62) noted the persistence of psychodynamic theories as a potential barrier, because many families perceive these theories as blaming. The findings on expression of emotion—the original basis for family psychoeducation—are often perceived similarly despite researchers' attempts to avoid implying blame (16,50).

Although the knowledge and underlying assumptions of individuals are important, they are only part of the picture. Wright (63) found that job and organizational factors were much better predictors of the frequency of mental health professionals' involvement with families than were professionals' attitudes. The clinician's work schedule and professional discipline were the strongest predictors, but other organizational factors posed barriers as well. Dissemination of the multiple-family psychoeducation group model developed by McFarlane and colleagues (64,59) has been hindered by a paucity of programmatic leadership, conflicts between the model's philosophy and typical agency practices, insuffi-

cient resources, and inadequate attention to human dynamics at the system level. For example, reasonable concerns about confidentiality may be seen as roadblocks to family involvement rather than as opportunities to create useful innovations (65). Similar barriers to implementation of family treatment approaches have been identified in studies in Italy (66).

Mental health professionals have also expressed concern about the cost and duration of structured family psychoeducation programs (67), even though medication and case management services for clients usually have to be continued for much longer periods than family programs. The lack of reimbursement for sessions with families that do not involve the mentally ill relative—a characteristic of many family psychoeducation programs—is a significant disincentive to providing such services. Caseloads are universally high, and staff's time is stretched thin. Therefore devoting substantial human resources to training, organizing, leading, and sustaining family psychoeducation is seen as a luxury (16). In such an atmosphere, horizons tend to be short. The long-term payoff of fewer crises and hospitalizations and lower total costs of treatment is overshadowed by immediate organizational crises or short-term goals (16).

Mental health authorities

At the health-system level, pressures to focus on outcomes, cost-effectiveness, and customer satisfaction seem in principle to favor the widespread adoption of family information and support interventions. However, other tenets of the current health care environment—such as the emphasis on short-term cost savings, technical rather than human-process-oriented remedies, and individual pathology—discourage clinicians from providing such services, which may be viewed as ancillary. At this level, it seems that the evidence for family psychoeducation has not been accepted. Many of the consumer- and program-level impediments we have mentioned are paralleled in the larger administrative systems: lack of awareness of evidence, ingrained assumptions about how care should be structured, and inadequate re-courcoc

Overcoming barriers to implementation

Research on technology transfer has identified four fundamental conditions that must be met for change to occur at the individual or system level: dissemination of knowledge, evaluation of programmatic impact, availability of resources, and efforts to address the human dynamics of resisting change (68). Implementation strategies must include clear, widespread communication of the models and of their benefits to all stakeholders. This communication must occur through channels that are accessible and acceptable to the various stakeholders (16), including families, consumers, providers, administrators, and policy makers. It must be accompanied by advocacy, training, and supervision or consultation initiatives to raise awareness and support at all organizational levels (69).

The consumer and family members

At the level of the individual consumer and members of his or her family, effective treatment models include strategies for overcoming barriers to participation, such as stigma and a sense of hopelessness. Such strategies include offering to hold sessions in the home of the client or family member; helping family members understand that the intervention is designed to improve the lives of everyone in the family, not just the patient; being flexible about scheduling family meetings; and providing education during the engagement process to destigmatize mental illness and engender hope (70,71).

Recent efforts to disseminate family psychoeducation in New York State, Los Angeles, Maine, and Illinois have illustrated clearly the importance of including clients and their families in the planning, adaptation, and eventual implementation of family psychoeducation (72). In New York, dissemination was initiated and sponsored by the state NAMI chapter (73). Dissemination in Maine and Illinois had dramatically different

outcomes, partly because NAMI's Maine chapter provided strong formal support for the effort in that state, whereas the effort in Illinois did not involve NAMI's Illinois chapters (73).

Experience and now some empirical data illustrate the need to include consumers and their families in efforts to disseminate family psychoeducation. The tension often encountered between some consumer advocacy groups and family advocacy organizations can be bridged by emphasizing the complementarity of the outcomes in family work: as consumers' symptoms are alleviated and their functioning improves, their families become more engaged in and satisfied with community life, and both the family burden and medical illness decrease (22,74,75).

Clinicians and program administrators

Among professionals working in community mental health services, awareness and evidence, although necessary, are often not sufficient for adoption of new programs. Although interventions must adhere to parameters of the family psychoeducation model if good client and family outcomes are to be achieved, they also have to be responsive to local organizational and community cultures. Engagement and implementation strategies, as well as the interventions themselves, must be tailored to local and cultural characteristics, workload and other stresses faced by clinicians and agencies, particular diagnoses, relationships, the duration of illness and disability, and whether the client is currently receiving medical treatment (50,76,77).

Perhaps even more critical to the adoption of family psychoeducation is the need to match both administrative support and expectations for evidence-based practice with a rationale and explication of the advantages of this treatment approach that are meaningful to clinicians. Advantages can include avoidance of crises, more efficient case management, gratitude from families and consumers, and a more interesting, invigorating work environment for clinicians. Recent studies have shown that on the

whole, knowledge about empirical advantages of family psychoeducation, such as reductions in relapse and rehospitalization rates, carry almost no weight in convincing working clinicians to change their attitudes toward families and adopt new clinical practices (73).

Consensus building among agency staff and directors—including a wide range of concerned parties—in a process of planning from the bottom up is critical but must be tailored to address local operational barriers and contrary beliefs. In addition, successful implementation of family psychoeducation has required ongoing supervision, operational consultation, and general support. In a sense, these characteristics help to build consensus on an ongoing basis. For example, the PORT found that it was possible to change current practice by providing a high level of technical assistance and a supportive environment that reflected staff agreement with the principles and philosophy of the new program (67). The recent dissemination of a family psychoeducation program in Los Angeles County succeeded because of the persistent advocacy of the local NAMI group, the support of top management, a nine-month training period, the high aptitude and strong commitment of the trainees, and the skill of the trainer (72).

Mental health authorities and government

Although it is tempting to assume that implementation of family psychoeducation could be mandated centrally by state mental health authorities, experience suggests that a more complex approach is required. Dissemination of a family psychoeducation program in New York State succeeded partly because of a partnership between the state, the NAMI affiliate, and an academic center. Unfortunately, the state's mental health authority abruptly terminated this large dissemination program before a widespread impact could be made. Maine's recent success was initiated by a state trade association of mental health centers and services, with support from but little involvement by the state mental health authority, which recently began exploring a formal partnership to continue and deepen this largely successful effort. A simultaneous effort in Illinois, initiated by the state authority but distinctly lacking consensus among center directors or the state NAMI chapter, has been less successful (73). One state that has had some success is New Jersey, which was able to disseminate family psychoeducation by setting expectations and requirements at the state level.

With the exception of the New Jersey effort, experience suggests that the most promising strategy is one in which provider organizations take the initiative with support from consumer and family organizations, the state mental health authority, and the key insurance payers. Appropriate reimbursement for family psychoeducation will follow. Experience also suggests that several years of consistent effort and ongoing monitoring are required for success. Fortunately, this process is not necessarily an expensive one: Maine implemented its family psychoeducation program in more than 90 percent of agencies for about 25 cents per capita over four years, including evaluation costs. The principal costs are in human effort, especially the effort required to overcome resistance to change.

Delivery of services to families must be subject to accountability and tracking. Although many states encourage the delivery of services to families, few monitor such services or make funding contingent on the services being delivered (78). One system-level option is for mental health centers to create a position for an adult family intervention coordinator, who would serve as the contact person for interventions, facilitate communication between staff and families, supervise clinicians, and monitor fidelity (79).

Family-to-Family Education Program

In the absence of family psychoeducation programs, voluntary peer-led family education programs have developed, epitomized by NAMI's Family-to-Family Education Program (FFEP) (14,80–82). FFEP is currently available in 41 states, many of which have waiting lists. FFEP and other mutual-assistance family programs are organized and led by trained volunteers from families of persons who have mental illness.

These community programs are offered regardless of the mentally ill person's treatment status. They tend to be brief—for example, 12 weeks for FFEP—and mix families of persons with various diagnoses, although they focus on persons with schizophrenia or bipolar disorder. On the basis of a trauma-and-recovery model of a family's experience in coping with mental illness, FFEP merges education with specific support mechanisms to help families through the various stages of comprehending and coping with a family member's mental illness (14). The program focuses first on outcomes of family members and their well-being, although benefits to the patient are also considered to be important (50).

Uncontrolled research on FFEP and its predecessor, Journey of Hope, suggests that the program increases the participants' knowledge about the causes and treatment of mental illness, their understanding of the mental health system, and their well-being (13). In a prospective, naturalistic study, FFEP participants reported that they had significantly less displeasure and concern about members of their family who had mental illness and significantly more empowerment at the family, community, and service-system levels after they had completed the program (83). Benefits observed at the end of the program had been sustained six months after the intervention. Preliminary results from a second ongoing study with a waiting-list control design have revealed similar findings.

Although FFEP currently lacks rigorous scientific evidence of efficacy in improving clinical or functional outcomes of persons who have mental illness, it shows considerable promise for improving the well-being of family members. In recent research and practice, attempts have been made to optimize the clinical opportunities provided by family psychoeducation and peer-based programs such as FFEP by developing partnerships between the two strate-gies. For example, family psychoeducation programs have used FFEP teachers as leaders, and participation in FFEP has facilitated eventual participation in family psychoeducation.

Conclusions

The efficacy and effectiveness of family psychoeducation as an evidence-based practice have been established. To date, the use of family psychoeducation in routine clinical practice is alarmingly limited. Research has recently begun to develop dissemination interventions targeted at the programmatic and organizational levels, with some success. Ongoing research must continue to develop practical and low-cost strategies to introduce and sustain family psychoeducation in typical practice settings. Basic research that identifies the barriers to implementing family psychoeducation in various clinical settings is also needed—for example, the impact of clinicians' attitudes, geographic factors, funding, disconnection of patients from family members, and stigma—as well as the extent to which variations in these factors mediate the outcomes of educational interventions.

Dissemination could also be facilitated by further exploring the integration of family psychoeducation with psychosocial interventions—such as assertive community treatment, supported employment, and social skills training—and other evidence-based cognitive-behavioral strategies for improving the treatment outcomes of persons with mental illness. Promising efforts have combined the energy, enthusiasm, and expertise of grassroots family organizations such as NAMI with professional and clinical programs. ◆

References

1. Cochrane JJ, Goering PN, Rogers JM: The mental health of informal caregivers in Ontario: an epidemiological survey. American Journal of Public Health 87:2002–2008, 1997

2. Leff J: Working with the families of schizophrenic patients. British Journal of Psychiatry Supplement 23(Apr):71–76, 1994

3. Schene AH, van Wijngaarden B, Koeter MWJ: Family caregiving in schizophrenia: domains and distress. Schizophrenia Bulletin 24:609–618, 1998

4. McFarlane WR, Lukens EP, Link B, et al:

Multiple-family groups and psychoeducation in the treatment of schizophrenia. Archives of General Psychiatry 52:679–687, 1995

5. Adamec C: How to Live With a Mentally Ill Person. New York, Wiley, 1996

6. Marsh DT, Johnson DL: The family experience of mental illness: implications for intervention. Professional Psychology: Research and Practice 28:229–237, 1997

7. Marsh DT: Families and Mental Illness: New Directions in Professional Practice. New York, Praeger, 1992

8. Anderson CM, Reiss DJ, Hogarty GE: Schizophrenia and the Family. New York, Guilford, 1986

9. Falloon IRH, Boyd JL, McGill CW: Family Care of Schizophrenia: A Problem-Solving Approach to the Treatment of Mental Illness. New York, Guilford, 1984

10. Marsh DT: A Family-Focused Approach to Serious Mental Illness: Empirically Supported Interventions. Sarasota, Fla, Professional Resource Press, 2001

11. Mannion E: Training Manual for the Implementation of Family Education in the Adult Mental Health System of Berks County, PA. Philadelphia, University of Pennsylvania Center for Mental Health Policy and Services Research, 2000

12. Amenson C: Schizophrenia: A Family Education Curriculum. Pasadena, Calif, Pacific Clinics Institute, 1998

13. Pickett-Schenk SA, Cook JA, Laris A: Journey of Hope program outcomes. Community Mental Health Journal 36:413–424, 2000

14. Burland JF: Family-to-Family: a trauma and recovery model of family education. New Directions for Mental Health Services, no 77:33–44, 1998

15. Drake RE, Goldman HH, Leff HS, et al: Implementing evidence-based practices in routine mental health service settings. Psychiatric Services 52:179–182, 2001

16. Families as Partners in Care: A Document Developed to Launch a Strategy for the Implementation of Programs of Family Education, Training, and Support. Toronto, World Schizophrenia Fellowship, 1998

17. Penn LD, Mueser KT: Research update on the psychosocial treatment of schizophrenia. American Journal of Psychiatry 153:607–617, 1996

18. Dixon LB, Lehman AF: Family interventions for schizophrenia. Schizophrenia Bulletin 21:631–643, 1995

19. Lam DH, Kuipers L, Leff JP: Family work with patients suffering from schizophrenia: the impact of training on psychiatric nurses' attitude and knowledge. Journal of Advanced Nursing 18:233–237, 1993

20. Falloon IRH, Held T, Coverdale JH, et al: Psychosocial interventions for schizophrenia: a review of long-term benefits of international studies. Psychiatric Rehabilitation Skills 3:268–290, 1999

21. Falloon IRH, Pederson J: Family management in the prevention of morbidity of schizophrenia: the adjustment family unit. British Journal of Psychiatry 147:156–163, 1985

22. McFarlane WR, Dushay R, Statsny P, et al: A comparison of two levels of family-aided assertive community treatment. Psychiatric Services 47:744–750, 1996

23. Cardin VA, McGill CW, Falloon IRH: An economic analysis: costs, benefits, and effectiveness, in Family Management of Schizophrenia. Edited by Falloon IRH. Baltimore, Johns Hopkins University Press, 1986

24. Tarrier N, Lowson K, Barrowclough C: Some aspects of family interventions in schizophrenia: II. financial considerations. British Journal of Psychiatry 159:481–484, 1991

25. Lehman AF, Steinwachs DM: At issue: translating research into practice: the Schizophrenia Patient Outcomes Research Team (PORT) treatment recommendations. Schizophrenia Bulletin 24:1–9, 1998

26. American Psychiatric Association Practice Guidelines for the Treatment of Schizophrenia. Washington, DC, American Psychiatric Association, 1997

27. Treatment of schizophrenia: the expert consensus panel for schizophrenia. Journal of Clinical Psychiatry 57(suppl 12B):3–58, 1996

28. Weiden PJ, Scheifler PL, McEvoy JP, et al: Expert consensus treatment guidelines for schizophrenia: a guide for patients and families. Journal of Clinical Psychiatry 60(suppl 11):73–80, 1999

29. Coursey RD, Curtis L, Marsh D, et al: Competencies for direct service staff members who work with adults with severe mental illness in outpatient public mental health managed care systems. Psychiatric Rehabilitation Journal 23:370–377, 2000

30. Coursey RD, Curtis L, Marsh D, et al: Competencies for direct service staff members who work with adults with severe mental illness: specific knowledge, attitudes, skills, and bibliography. Psychiatric Rehabilitation Journal 23:378–392, 2000

31. Greenberg JS, Greenley JR, Kim HW: The provision of mental health services to families of persons with serious mental illness. Research in Community and Mental Health 8:181–204, 1995

32. Cuijpers P: The effects of family interventions on relatives' burden: a meta-analysis. Journal of Mental Health 8:275–285, 1999

33. Clarkin JF, Carpenter D, Hull J, et al: Effects of psychoeducational intervention for married patients with bipolar disorder and their spouses. Psychiatric Services 49:531–533, 1998

34. Miklowitz D, Goldstein M: Bipolar Disorder: A Family-Focused Treatment Approach. New York, Guilford, 1997

35. Moltz D: Bipolar disorder and the family: an integrative model. Family Process 32:409–423, 1993

36. Parikh SV, Kusumakar V, Haslam DR, et al: Psychosocial interventions as an adjunct to pharmacotherapy in bipolar disorder. Canadian Journal of Psychiatry 42(suppl 2):74S–78S, 1997

37. Miklowitz DJ, Simoneau TL, George EL, et al: Family-focused treatment of bipolar disorder: one-year effects of a psychoeducational program in conjunction with pharmacotherapy. Biological Psychiatry 48:582–592, 2000

38. Simoneau TL, Miklowitz DJ, Richards JA, et al: Bipolar disorder and family communication: the effects of a psychoeducational treatment program. Journal of Abnormal Psychology 108:588–597, 1999

39. Emanuels-Zuurveen L, Emmelkamp PM: Individual behavioural-cognitive therapy: V. marital therapy for depression in maritally distressed couples. British Journal of Psychiatry 169:181–188, 1996

40. Emanuels-Zuurveen L, Emmelkamp PM: Spouse-aided therapy with depressed patients. Behavior Modification 21:62–77, 1997

41. Leff JL, Vearnals S, Brewin CR, et al: The London Depression Intervention Trial: randomised controlled trial of antidepressants v couple therapy in the treatment and maintenance of people with depression living with a partner: clinical outcome and costs. British Journal of Psychiatry 177:95–100, 2000

42. Van Noppen B: Multi-family behavioral treatment (MFBT) for OCD crisis intervention and time-limited treatment. Crisis Intervention and Time-Limited Treatment 5:3–24, 1999

43. Geist R, Heinmaa M, Stephens D, et al: Comparison of family therapy and family group psychoeducation in adolescents with anorexia nervosa. Canadian Journal of Psychiatry 45:173–178, 2000

44. Gunderson JG, Berkowitz C, Ruizsancho A: Families of borderline patients: a psychoeducational approach. Bulletin of the Menninger Clinic 61:446–457, 1997

45. Gonzalez S, Steinglass P, Reiss D: Putting the illness in its place: discussion groups for families with chronic medical illnesses. Family Process 28:69–87, 1989

46. Schooler NR, Keith SJ, Severe JB, et al: Relapse and rehospitalization during maintenance treatment of schizophrenia: the effects of dose reduction and family treatment. Archives of General Psychiatry 54:453–463, 1997

47. Stein LL, Santos AB: Assertive Community Treatment of Persons With Severe Mental Illness. New York, Norton, 1998

48. Bond GR, Becker DR, Drake RE, et al: Implementing supported employment as an evidenced-based practice. Psychiatric Services 52:313–322, 2001

49. McFarlane WR, Dushay RA, Deakins S, et al: Employment outcomes in family-aided assertive community treatment. American Journal of Orthopsychiatry 70:203–214, 2000

50. Solomon P: Moving from psychoeducation

to family education for families of adults with serious mental illness. Psychiatric Services 47:1364–1370, 1996

51. Solomon P, Draine JE, Mannion E: The impact of individualized consultation and group workshop family education interventions on ill relative outcomes. Journal of Nervous and Mental Disease 184:252–255, 1996

52. Solomon P, Draine J, Mannion E, et al: Effectiveness of two models of brief family education: retention of gains by family members of adults with serious mental illness. American Journal of Orthopsychiatry 67:177–186, 1997

53. Cañive JM, Sanz-Fuentenebro J, Vazquez C, et al: Family psychoeducational support groups in Spain: parents' distress and burden at nine-month follow-up. Annals of Clinical Psychiatry 8:71–79, 1996

54. Telles C, Karno M, Mintz J, et al: Immigrant families coping with schizophrenia: behavioral family intervention v case management with a low-income Spanish-speaking population. British Journal of Psychiatry 167:473–479, 1995

55. Xiang MG, Ran MS, Li SG: A controlled evaluation of psychoeducational family intervention in a rural Chinese community. British Journal of Psychiatry 165:544–548, 1994

56. Xiong W, Phillips MR, Hu X, et al: Family-based intervention for schizophrenic patients in China: a randomized controlled trial. British Journal of Psychiatry 165:239–247, 1994

57. Zhang M, Wang M, Li J, et al: Randomized-control trial of family intervention for 78 first-episode male schizophrenic patients: an 18-month study in Suzhou, Jiangsu. British Journal of Psychiatry 165(suppl 24):96–102, 1994

58. Lefley HP: Impact of mental illness on families and carers, in Textbook of Community Psychiatry. Edited by Thornicroft G, Szmukler G. London, Oxford University Press, 2001

59. McFarlane WR, Dunne E, Lukens E: From research to clinical practice: dissemination of New York State's family psychoeducation project. Hospital and Community Psychiatry 44:265–270, 1993

60. Gallagher SK, Mechanic D: Living with the mentally ill: effects on the health and functioning of other household members. Social Science and Medicine 42:1691–1701, 1996

61. Mueser KT, Webb C, Pfeiffer M, et al: Family burden of schizophrenia and bipolar disorder: perceptions of relatives and professionals. Psychiatric Services 47:507–511, 1996

62. Bergmark T. Models of family support in Sweden: from mistreatment to understanding. New Directions in Mental Health Services 62:71–77, 1994

63. Wright ER: The impact of organizational factors on mental health professionals' involvement with families. Psychiatric Services 48:921–927, 1997

64. Dixon L, McFarlane W, Hornby H, et al: Dissemination of family psychoeducation: the importance of consensus building. Schizophrenia Research 36:339, 1999

65. Bogart T, Solomon P: Procedures to share treatment information among mental health providers, consumer, and families. Psychiatric Services 50:1321–1325, 2000

66. Falloon IRH, Casacchia M, Lussetti M, et al: The development of cognitive-behavioural therapies within Italian mental health services. International Journal of Mental Health 28:60–67, 1999

67. Dixon L, Lyles A, Scott J, et al: Services to families of adults with schizophrenia: from treatment recommendations to dissemination. Psychiatric Services 50:233–238, 1999

68. Backer T: Drug Abuse Technology Transfer. Rockville, Md, National Institute on Drug Abuse, 1991

69. McFarlane WR: Multiple-family groups and psychoeducation in the treatment of schizophrenia. New Directions for Mental Health Services, no 62:13–22, 1994

70. Mueser KT, Glynn SM: Behavioral Family Therapy for Psychiatric Disorders. Oakland, Calif, New Harbinger, 1999

71. Tarrier N: Some aspects of family interventions in schizophrenia: I. adherence to intervention programmes. British Journal of Psychiatry 159:475–480, 1991

72. Amenson CS, Liberman RP: Dissemination of educational classes for families of

adults with schizophrenia. Psychiatric Services 52:589–592, 2001

73. McFarlane WR, McNary S, Dixon L, et al: Predictors of dissemination of family psychoeducation in community mental health centers in Maine and Illinois. Psychiatric Services, 52:935–942, 2001

74. Falloon IRH, Falloon NCH, Lussetti M: Integrated Mental Health Care: A Guidebook for Consumers. Perugia, Italy, Optimal Treatment Project, 1997

75. Dyck DG, Short RA, Hendry M, et al: Management of negative symptoms among patients with schizophrenia attending multiple-family groups. Psychiatric Services 51:513–519, 2000

76. Guarnaccia P, Parra P: Ethnicity, social status, and families' experiences of caring for a mentally ill family member. Community Mental Health Journal 32:243–260, 1996

77. Jordan C, Lewellen A, Vandiver V: Psychoeducation for minority families: a social-work perspective. International Journal of Mental Health 23(4):27–43, 1995

78. Dixon L, Goldman HH, Hirad A: State policy and funding of services to families of adults with serious and persistent mental illness. Psychiatric Services 50:551–552, 1999

79. Mueser KT, Fox L: Family-friendly services: a modest proposal [letter]. Psychiatric Services 51:1452, 2000

80. Solomon P, Draine J, Mannion E: The impact of individualized consultation and group workshop family education interventions in ill relative outcomes. Journal of Nervous and Mental Disease 184:252–255, 1996

81. Solomon P, Draine J, Mannion E, et al: Impact of brief family psychoeducation on self-efficacy. Schizophrenia Bulletin 22:41–50, 1996

82. Solomon P: Interventions for families of individuals with schizophrenia: maximizing outcomes for their relatives. Disease Management and Health Outcomes 8:211–221, 2000

83. Dixon L, Stewart B, Burland J, et al: Pilot study of the effectiveness of the Family-to-Family Education Program. Psychiatric Services 52:965–967, 2001

Evidence-Based Pharmacologic Treatment for People With Severe Mental Illness: A Focus on Guidelines and Algorithms

Thomas A. Mellman, M.D.
Alexander L. Miller, M.D.
Ellen M. Weissman, M.D.
M. Lynn Crismon, Pharm.D.
Susan M. Essock, Ph.D.
Stephen R. Marder, M.D.

Medication treatment of severe mental illness has been advanced and complicated by the introduction of numerous therapeutic agents. Practice guidelines based on research evidence have been developed to help clinicians make complex decisions. Studies of usual care suggest an important potential role for guidelines in improving the quality of medication treatment for people with severe mental illness. The authors review current evidence-based guidelines for medication treatment of persons with severe mental illness. Four categories of guidelines are described: recommendations, comprehensive treatment options, medication algorithms, and expert consensus. The authors note that more research is needed on optimal next-step strategies and the treatment of patients with comorbidity and other complicating problems. They discuss barriers to the implementation of guidelines, and they observe that the potential of guidelines and algorithms to promote evidence-based medication treatment for persons with severe mental illness depends on refinement of tools, progress in research, and cooperation of physicians, nonphysician clinicians, administrators, and consumers and family members.

In psychiatry, as in all branches of medicine, an ever-expanding range of therapeutic options is being created. One response to this evolving complexity has been the development of guidelines intended to inform and influence clinical practice. A proximal goal of practice guidelines is to promote the use of effective therapeutic interventions and reduce inappropriate variation in clinical practice. Guideline implementation is also expected to improve outcomes and facilitate cost management (1).

Most practice guidelines incorporate and summarize research evidence that supports their recommendations. It is a formidable challenge for busy clinicians to keep up with the high volume of research findings. Thus an additional purpose of practice guidelines is to disseminate research findings of direct relevance to clinical practice. At the systems level, practice guidelines can facilitate a systematic approach to medication management of chronic illnesses across treatment venues and prescribers.

The complexity of practice, the volume of research findings, and the advent of guidelines are trends that have become particularly germane to pharmacologic treatment of people with severe mental illness. During the past 15 years, more than ten new antipsychotic and antidepressant medications have been approved for use in the United States, and several new mood stabilizers have been identified. The comparatively favorable safety and side-effect profiles of these agents as well as their putative therapeutic advantages have raised expectations for improved outcomes with psychiatric medications.

The availability of these medications may also contribute to greater comfort with prescription of combinations of psychotropic medications. The proliferation of new agents and the resulting increase in potential medication combinations, along with elevated treatment goals, all add to the importance and challenge of defining and implementing evidence-based psychopharmacologic practice.

Higher costs associated with new medications and polypharmacy are a

Dr. Mellman is associate professor of psychiatry at the Dartmouth Medical School, Dartmouth-Hitchcock Medical Center, Department of Psychiatry, One Medical Center Drive, Lebanon, New Hampshire 03756 (e-mail, mellman@dartmouth.edu). Dr. Miller is professor of psychiatry at the University of Texas Health Science Center at San Antonio. Dr. Weissman is assistant professor of psychiatry and Dr. Essock is professor of psychiatry at Mount Sinai School of Medicine in New York City. Dr. Crismon is professor at the University of Texas College of Pharmacy in Austin. Dr. Marder is professor of psychiatry at the University of California at Los Angeles School of Medicine. This article was originally published in the May 2001 issue of Psychiatric Services.

growing concern for mental health administrators, policy makers, consumers and their families, and the public. The question of how the implementation of guidelines would influence medication costs and other costs related to treatment and the impact of illness is currently unanswered. Use of guidelines may reduce costs by eliminating ineffective practices. The more likely benefit of guidelines is in producing greater value per health care dollar.

In this article we discuss guidelines and algorithms as a means of addressing the complexity of pharmacologic treatment of people with severe mental illnesses and disseminating relevant research findings. Our definition of severe mental illness includes psychotic disorders, mood disorders, and certain anxiety disorders—panic disorder, posttraumatic stress disorder, and obsessive-compulsive disorder. This definition is in keeping with the substantial impairment and chronicity associated with these disorders (2,3) and the range of problems typically addressed with medication treatment in mental health settings. We do not review important work on the screening and management of anxiety and depression in primary care settings. We describe relevant guidelines and discuss the nature and limitations of the supporting evidence. We then explore barriers to guideline implementation and critical components of guidelines and make recommendations for facilitating and furthering evidence-based practices in the pharmacologic treatment of people with severe mental illnesses.

Overview of current guidelines and algorithms

The current guidelines that address pharmacologic treatment of severe mental illness fall into one of four categories, according to their scope and the stringency with which they rely on empirical evidence: recommendations, comprehensive treatment options, medication algorithms, and expert consensus. All of these categories are distinct from specific, highly proscriptive protocols that might be in place in some clinical settings. Although the recommended therapeutic options tend to be consistent across the existing guidelines, they differ in scope.

Recommendations

The first category, recommendations, is exemplified by the Patient Outcomes Research Team (PORT) treatment recommendations for schizophrenia (4). The development of the PORT recommendations was initially sponsored by the U.S. Agency for Health Care Policy and Research. The PORT project was regionally based; however, three research centers participated. Methods for developing the recommendations included a literature review followed by reviews of additional experts. Rigorous requirements were established for evidence to support revision.

The PORT recommendations are supported by "substantial evidence of efficacy," and the strength of specific supporting evidence is documented in the guidelines. The PORT recommendations address antipsychotic and adjunctive medications, electroconvulsive therapy (ECT), and several psychosocial interventions. Most PORT recommendations are definitive, as embodied in statements such as "antipsychotic medications, other than clozapine, should be used as first-line treatment." The PORT guidelines also recommend use of conventional doses and maintenance on continuing treatment for at least a year for people who respond to treatment. Certain practices, such as "loading" medication treatment with "massive" doses, are discouraged. Clozapine is advocated as an approach for people who have not experienced adequate reduction in symptoms with previous antipsychotic medication treatment.

Comprehensive treatment options

Practice guidelines in the second category have been developed predominantly by professional organizations. These guidelines are comprehensive in the scope of therapeutic options presented. Thresholds for the strength of evidence required to support recommended treatment options tend to be less stringent than for the PORT treatment recommendations, and these guidelines, accordingly, are less proscriptive. The

methods for developing these guidelines overlap with those described for PORT and include expert working groups, literature reviews, secondary expert review, and revision. Guidelines developed through professional organizations ultimately require organizational approval.

Pharmacologic treatment is addressed in detail by practice guidelines for the treatment of patients with bipolar disorder (5), schizophrenia (6), major depressive disorder (7), and panic disorder (8) developed by the American Psychiatric Association (APA) and practice guidelines for the treatment of posttraumatic stress disorder (PTSD) developed by the International Society for Traumatic Stress Studies (ISTSS) (9). Except for schizophrenia and bipolar disorder, specific psychotherapies are presented as first-line alternatives to medication. Newer medications tend to be favored for initial intervention; lithium for bipolar disorder is the most notable exception.

The recently revised APA depression treatment guidelines also endorse as first-line therapeutic options the tricyclic antidepressants desipramine and nortriptyline, along with selective serotonin reuptake inhibitors (SSRIs) and antidepressants that have been marketed more recently (6). The ISTSS guidelines for PTSD give the strongest endorsement to SSRIs as a first-line medication option on the basis of data supporting their effectiveness and limited research evaluation of alternative treatments (9). For bipolar illness, lithium or the anticonvulsant valproate are endorsed for first-line therapy (5).

Algorithms

An algorithm is a rule or set of rules that is applied to solving a problem. Medication algorithms are a subset of practice guidelines. They are distinguished by an exclusive focus on medications and by a more step-by-step approach to clinical decisions. The Texas Medication Algorithm Project (TMAP) constitutes the most extensive and comprehensive development and implementation to date of medication algorithms for persons with serious mental illness. Current projects address the treatment of schizophrenia, bipolar disorder, and major depression.

TMAP was initiated by the Texas Department of Mental Health and Mental Retardation in collaboration with a consortium of Texas academic medical centers. The development of the TMAP algorithms incorporated expert panels, literature review, and consensus conferences. Development has also incorporated consumer input and revisions solicited from academic and nonacademic clinicians. Field-testing to evaluate clinical and economic impact is under way, principally in the public mental health system of the state of Texas (10,11).

The Texas Implementation of Medication Algorithms (TIMA) is the practical, clinician-targeted implementation of TMAP. TIMA and TMAP user manuals are available on the Internet (www.mhmr.state.tx.us/centraloffice/medicaldirector/tima or tmap), and outlines and summaries have been presented in the literature. All the presentations feature flow diagrams that provide recommendations linked to specific stages of treatment. Like other practice guidelines described in this paper, TMAP recommends a range of stage 1, or first-line, treatment initiation strategies without prioritizing among them. For the treatment of unipolar, nonpsychotic major depression, stage 1 options are the "new-generation" antidepressants (11); for mania, stage 1 options are lithium and one of two anticonvulsants (12). All of the atypical or novel antipsychotics other than clozapine are recommended for the initial treatment of schizophrenia (13). Adequate response dictates continuation of stage 1 therapy.

The most notable aspect of TMAP may be the degree of elaboration of stepwise strategies for partial response, nonresponse, or medication intolerance. Stage 2 and subsequent stages comprise sequences of alternative medication treatment options. Staging for inadequate responders ultimately leads to recommendations such as clozapine, ECT, or combinations of medications. Initial stages of treatment usually feature monotherapy, except for the treatment of bipolar and psychotic depression. In addition to presenting the algorithms, TIMA and TMAP documents include information on dosing, side-effect profiles, and the tools used for assessment and monitoring as well as consumer education material.

Expert consensus guidelines

The fourth category, expert consensus guidelines, is quite distinct from the categories previously considered. Recommendations are based on the results of surveying a relatively broad array of experts in the treatment of the condition in question and do not rely directly on analysis of the research literature. The stated purpose of this approach is to supplement "the first generation of treatment guidelines," and its rationale is that research literature sometimes does not adequately address critical points for treatment decisions (14). Expert consensus guidelines for the treatment of schizophrenia (15), bipolar disorder (16), obsessive-compulsive disorder (17), agitation in older persons with dementia (18), and PTSD (19) have been published as supplements in journals and are available on the Internet (www.psychguides.com). Statistical results of questionnaire-based surveys addressing the appropriateness of interventions for different stages of treatment are presented, along with guidelines synthesized from the survey results.

Other efforts

Additional examples that illustrate the scope of emerging guidelines relevant to pharmacologic treatment in psychiatry include the recent implementation of guidelines by the U.S. Department of Veterans Affairs for screening, referring, and managing depression among persons with and without PTSD and substance abuse and for treating psychosis (see www.va.gov for more information). The Canadian Psychiatric Association has developed practice guidelines for the treatment of schizophrenia that have an emphasis similar to that of the APA guidelines (20). Guidelines developed by the American Academy of Child and Adolescent Psychia-

try for the treatment of disorders presenting in children and adolescents address therapeutic modalities comprehensively and provide recommendations about the role of medication (21). Texas now has a children's medication algorithm project (CMAP) that addresses the use of medication for childhood and adolescent depression and attention-deficit hyperactivity disorder and co-morbid disorders (22).

Nature and limitations of the evidence

Most guideline documents include a critical appraisal of the quality of supporting evidence for each recommendation. The highest levels of confidence are assigned to recommendations supported by multiple randomized controlled clinical trials. Gradations of confidence are generally rated on considerations that include the number and quality of research studies and the consistency of findings.

Recommendations made with high confidence are those that are based on evidence supporting the efficacy of first-line acute treatments for schizophrenia, mood disorders, and most anxiety disorders as well as on evidence supporting the role in relapse prevention of continuation of these treatments. In recent guidelines, the newer psychotropic agents are preferred as first-line agents. Their use is justified principally by their safety and tolerability profiles. First-line use of the newer antipsychotic medications may also offer advantages in the areas of negative symptoms and cognition. However, as experience with newer agents has accumulated, their advantages have been debated, and unforeseen risks, such as weight gain, have been identified. As Miller and associates concluded in their review (23), clozapine is not considered a first-line option because of safety concerns and monitoring requirements.

Recommendations for next-step strategies for patients who respond only partially or who do not respond to these agents and recommendations for treating patients with complex comorbidity often rely on more limited research evidence, such as open studies and case series, and on expert opinion. Most recommendations for treatment-resistant patients with severe mental illness are not guided by a strong research base. There are a few notable exceptions. The utility of clozapine for treating persons with schizophrenia who do not respond adequately to traditional antipsychotic agents has been established by controlled trials that featured prospective determination of treatment nonresponsiveness (24).

Similar studies were not required for the approval of risperidone, olanzapine, and quetiapine by the U.S. Food and Drug Administration (FDA), and such studies are just beginning to appear in the literature. Available studies of these novel antipsychotic medications provide more limited support (25) or are not supportive (26) of efficacy when the initial treatment strategy is ineffective. In addition, in these studies, treatment refractoriness is usually defined in the context of traditional antipsychotic medications. Because atypical antipsychotics are now being used as first-line agents, research is needed to evaluate next-step strategies for patients who are treatment resistant to atypical antipsychotics.

For patients with depression who are unresponsive or partially responsive to initial treatment, extensive evidence supports a reasonable probability that patients who have not adequately responded to or tolerated some agents will respond to others (27). The best-studied medication strategy for refractory major depression other than switching agents is lithium augmentation—the addition of lithium to existing treatment. The TMAP algorithms recommend lithium augmentation before augmentation with other medications and before combination strategies (11). It is not known how lithium augmentation compares with alternative strategies that may currently be more popular, such as the addition of bupropion to an SSRI, an intervention that is mainly supported by a theoretical rationale and uncontrolled observations (28).

Some widely used strategies for augmenting antidepressant response have not withstood the test of a randomized controlled trial (29,30).

Other next-step strategies for the treatment of mood disorders that are supported by reasonable evidence include combinations of mood stabilizers in bipolar disorder (31) and ECT. ECT, which is considered more invasive than pharmacologic treatment, is a well-established approach to treatment-refractory mood disorders (32).

There are other categories of severe mental illness in which medication treatment is often used but is generally understudied. For example, research evaluating medication treatment for PTSD is limited but is gaining momentum. A large study that showed the efficacy of sertraline, an SSRI, in the treatment of PTSD recently led to FDA approval of the addition of PTSD to sertraline's on-label indications (33). Few studies have examined second-line medication strategies and treatment of comorbid presentations that would be highly relevant to clinical practice. To our knowledge, some evidence has not yet been synthesized into guidelines. This evidence supports the apparently common practice of pharmacologically targeting mood symptoms and impulsivity in borderline and other severe personality disorders (34,35). The rationale for much of the prescribing for patients with a dual diagnosis—severe mental illness co-occurring with a substance use disorder—is extrapolated from studies of non-substance-abusing populations. Studies that specifically address efficacy and safety in younger populations are sorely needed as the use of psychotropic medications by children and adolescents increases (36).

Conformance of usual care

We are unaware of any published reports showing the impact on treatment outcomes of implementing pharmacologic treatment guidelines in mental health settings. However, a few studies have evaluated how closely usual care resembles that suggested by guideline recommendations. The PORT project included a survey of usual care for people with schizophrenia from geographically diverse public-sector settings. The rates at which usual practice

conformed to medication recommendations varied. Antipsychotic medication was prescribed for 89 percent of inpatients and 92 percent of outpatients. Prescriptions conformed to dosage recommendations for 62 percent of the inpatients but for only 29 percent of the outpatients. Rates of use of adjunctive agents in cases in which they appear to have been therapeutically indicated ranged from 14 to 41 percent, depending on the setting (37).

Using criteria derived from the PORT recommendations, Young and associates (38) evaluated the adequacy of treatment for patients with schizophrenia in two large public mental health settings in Los Angeles in 1996. Inadequate treatment was defined as the presence of either significant side effects or unresolved symptoms, with no attempt made to alter medication therapy. At the two sites, the rates of inadequate treatment not attributable to patient factors were 28 percent and 16 percent, respectively. Use of the atypical or novel antipsychotics available at the time, clozapine and risperidone, was low (38).

Published studies, however, may not adequately capture the evolving landscape of pharmacologic treatment of severe mental illness. In keeping with recent guideline recommendations, treatment with atypical antipsychotic medications appears to be becoming the modal therapy for schizophrenia. A recent analysis used data from a Medicaid prescription database for the State of New Hampshire to identify a cohort of persons diagnosed as having schizophrenia (39). Prescription of atypical antipsychotic medications other than clozapine rose from 18 percent in 1995 to 54 percent in 1999. Clozapine use remained stable at 26 percent.

Concurrent prescription of two or more antipsychotic medications appeared to be a related trend (Clark RE, Mellman TA, Bartels SJ, et al, unpublished data, 2001). Rates of coprescription of antipsychotics rose from 6 percent in 1995 to 24 percent in 1999. In most cases, the duration of coprescription exceeded that expected during a straightforward medication switch—that is, cross-tapering. Further research is needed to provide an understanding of the course of treatment, the rationales, and the outcomes associated with this and other common forms of coprescription. The practice of coprescribing appears more common than would be expected if practice conformed to TMAP and other medication guidelines, which place combinations of antipsychotic medications at or near the last step of their recommendations.

Barriers to implementation

The findings discussed here suggest that implementation of guidelines can improve the quality of medication treatment for people with schizophrenia. It seems likely that the situation is similar for the usual treatment of other severe psychiatric disorders. For implementation to be successful, the effort must address potential barriers. Implementation of medication guidelines as well as barriers to implementation can be conceptually divided into two categories, systemic and individual.

At the systemic level, there must be a commitment to providing the tools necessary for guideline implementation. Practically speaking, this means providing the resources necessary to implement guidelines, such as ensuring that the recommended medications are on the formulary and that adequate time is provided for required assessments. In addition, documentation forms must be changed to facilitate recording and review of data used in making medication decisions, according to recommendations of the particular algorithm or guideline being implemented.

At the individual level, providers and patients must accept the guidelines as a reasonable approach to treatment that increases the likelihood of successful outcomes. Experience indicates that clinicians do not readily adhere to practice guidelines. Literature from nonpsychiatric medicine identifies barriers to clinicians' adherence, including lack of familiarity with guidelines, lack of agreement with or confidence in guidelines, practical limitations, and

practice inertia (39). Some clinicians may view guidelines as limiting their autonomy and creativity.

Barriers specific to clinical practice in psychiatry may complicate efforts to implement guidelines. Clinical histories that are used to "stage" patients in guideline-based treatment may be inaccurate when obtained from patients with severe mental illness, who may have symptoms that limit their ability to report their past treatment response adequately and for whom collateral informants may be lacking. Psychiatrists and other treatment staff as

It is

our experience

that practice within

appropriately constructed

guideline parameters readily

allows for consideration of

the individual and for

creative, individualized

treatment

planning.

well as patients and family members may be resistant to switching medications when the patient has a history of violence toward self or others or has gotten worse after previous medication changes. In many public-sector settings, patients who are considered stable by the treatment team continue to experience disabling symptoms. Because switching medications involves some risk of behavioral deterioration, treatment teams may forgo attempts to treat remaining symptoms in order to maintain the status quo.

Consumers and family members may fear that guidelines represent a

dehumanizing trend in health care that limits consideration of individuality. Although this concern is understandable, it is our experience that practice within appropriately constructed guideline parameters readily allows for consideration of the individual and for creative, individualized treatment planning. Guideline materials developed for consumers and their families can help them understand the rationale for current medication treatments and can serve as tools for initiating discussion of alternative considerations, thereby promoting shared decision making.

Critical components, current applications, and future issues

Discussions of evidence-based practice for nonpharmacologic treatments, including papers previously published and those projected for this series, emphasize implementation of underused effective practices. In contrast, pharmacologic treatment is accepted by most treatment providers and does not appear to be generally underused in the usual treatment of people with severe mental illness. Our emphasis is on using medication treatments that are evidence based and, whenever possible, on using them in sequences supported by research—that is, in conformance with the principles delineated in the guidelines and algorithms discussed in this paper.

What practices are needed for pharmacologic treatment for people with severe mental illnesses to conform to evidence-based principles? First, the clinician must make an accurate diagnosis and specify target symptoms and their initial severity. Second, the clinician should choose a medication and dosage range supported by the research evidence for the condition and target symptoms in question.

Third, the clinician should monitor changes in symptoms and the occurrence and tolerability of side effects. Determining adequacy of response and tolerance of side effects requires clinical judgment. Use of systematic rating instruments can make these determinations more precise. Determining appropriate thresholds to define adequate versus inadequate response is an important focus for continuing investigation.

Fourth, if medications are not tolerated well or symptoms do not respond after a trial of adequate duration, the clinician should consider strategies recommended by the illness-specific guidelines, such as raising the dosage, changing to another efficacious medication, or using an augmentation strategy. Fifth, similar approaches should be used to address co-occurring syndromes. Finally, the clinician must critically evaluate a patient's response to coadministered medication treatments—augmentation and combination strategies—and attempt to discontinue medications that have not improved the therapeutic response.

Although these principles may seem self-evident, it is not clear that they are routinely applied in many practice settings. The guidelines and algorithms present options for implementing evidence-based medication treatment. For example, the more proscriptive nature of the PORT guidelines leads to identification of treatments that do not conform to the usually recommended practices. In our view, given the present state of knowledge, it would not be appropriate to uniformly prohibit treatment approaches that do not conform to medication guidelines. Rather, many nonconforming practices might be held to greater scrutiny and standards for justification.

TMAP offers clinicians a convenient, comprehensive elaboration of next-step alternatives. The recent development of consumer-oriented materials is a promising approach to facilitating clinician-consumer dialogue and shared decision making (41).

The ultimate utility of guidelines and algorithms for promoting evidence-based medication treatment for people with severe mental illness depends on continuing refinement of guideline tools and progress in research. The likelihood that a busy clinician will refer to guideline material is greatly enhanced by efficient access to the information, ideally during the clinical encounter itself. The literature on guideline implementation in nonpsychiatric medicine suggests that computerized tools for tracking

clinical data and providing information offer advantages (41). The guidelines discussed in this paper address a range of problems from various perspectives. Tools that distill and synthesize key elements to educate clinicians and consumers should enhance guideline implementation. One worthwhile goal may be to integrate tools that apply to different disorders, which may facilitate comprehensive application of guidelines in public mental health settings.

Further development and dissemination of practical assessment and tracking tools would advance the implementation of evidence-based prescribing. Clinical decisions about changes in treatment after the initial intervention hinge on judgments of the adequacy of response. In research settings, diagnosis and therapeutic response are determined by systematic assessments with standardized tools. Although it is reasonable to apply some of the available rating instruments in clinical settings, others can be complicated and time-consuming. Research is needed to establish the validity of pared-down, clinician-friendly rating instruments. For assessment and tracking tools to be more widely accepted outside of research settings, they should not substantially increase, and ideally would decrease, the burden of documentation.

Research in these areas can better inform the next generation of guidelines and algorithms. We hope that the current prioritization of effectiveness research (42) will address the more critical gaps in current evidence.

Conclusions

The potential for guidelines to improve care ultimately depends on the acceptance and commitment of administrators, consumers, and members of the treatment team. Successful implementation of guidelines requires administrative support and motivated prescribers. Nonphysician members of the treatment team have a critical role in monitoring medication compliance, affecting patients' and families' attitudes toward changes in treatment, and providing critical feedback to prescribers about a patient's clinical state and treatment response. Consumers and their family

members must have an active role in discussing therapeutic options, initiating changes, and providing feedback about treatment response. Achieving the potential of improved quality of care through the use of medication guidelines founded on evidence-based practices requires collaboration between policy makers, administrators, providers, and consumers of psychiatric care. ♦

Acknowledgments

This work was supported by a grant from the Robert Wood Johnson Foundation and the Substance Abuse and Mental Health Services Administration. The authors thank Kara Comins, B.S., and Wendy Bayles-Dazet, R.N., for their assistance and Robert E. Drake, M.D., Ph.D., for comments on the manuscript.

References

1. Audet AM, Greenfield S, Field M: Medical practice guidelines: current activities and future directions. Annals Internal Medicine 30:709–714, 1999

2. Roy-Byrne PP, Stang P, Wittchen HU, et al: Lifetime panic-depression comorbidity in the National Comorbidity Survey: association with symptoms, impairment, course, and help-seeking. British Journal of Psychiatry 176:229–235, 2000

3. Kessler RC: Posttraumatic stress disorder: the burden to the individual and to society. Journal of Clinical Psychiatry 61(suppl 5):4–12, 2000

4. Lehman AF, Steinwachs DM: Translating research into practice: the Schizophrenia Patient Outcomes Research Team (PORT) treatment recommendations. Schizophrenia Bulletin 24:1–10, 1998

5. American Psychiatric Association Practice Guideline for the Treatment of Patients With Bipolar Disorder. American Journal of Psychiatry 151(Dec suppl):1–36, 1994

6. American Psychiatric Association Practice Guideline for the Treatment of Patients With Schizophrenia. American Journal of Psychiatry 154(Apr suppl):1–63, 1997

7. American Psychiatric Association Practice Guideline for the Treatment of Patients With Major Depressive Disorder. American Journal of Psychiatry 157:1–45, 2000

8. American Psychiatric Association Practice Guideline for the Treatment of Patients With Panic Disorder. American Journal of Psychiatry 155:1–34, 1998

9. Foa EB, Keane TM, Friedman MJ: Guidelines for treatment of PTSD. Journal of Traumatic Stress 13:539–588, 2000

10. Gilbert DA, Altshuler KZ, Rago WV, et al: Texas Medication Algorithm Project: definitions, rationale, and methods to develop

medication algorithms. Journal of Clinical Psychiatry 59:345–351, 1998

11. Crismon ML, Trivedi M, Pigott TA, et al: The Texas Medication Algorithm Project: report of the Texas consensus conference panel on medication treatment of major depressive disorder. Journal of Clinical Psychiatry 60:142–156, 1999

12. Suppes T, Brown A, Dennehy E, et al: Bipolar Disorders Module Guideline Procedures Manual. TMAP Procedural Manual 1:2, 1999. Available at www.mhmr.state.tx.us

13. Miller AL, Chiles JA, Chiles JK, et al: The Texas Medication Algorithm Project (TMAP) schizophrenia algorithms. Journal of Clinical Psychiatry 60:649–657, 1999

14. Frances F, Kahn D, Carpenter D, et al: The Expert Consensus Practice Guideline Project: a new method of establishing best practice. Journal of Practicing Behavioral Health 5:295–306, 1996

15. McEvoy J, Weiden P, Smith T, et al (eds): The Expert Consensus Guideline Series: treatment of schizophrenia. Journal of Clinical Psychiatry 57(suppl 12B):1–58, 1996

16. Kahn D, Carpenter D, Docherty J, et al (eds): The Expert Consensus Guideline Series: treatment of bipolar disorder. Journal of Clinical Psychiatry 57(suppl 12A):1–88, 1996

17. March JS, Frances A, Carpenter D, et al (eds): The Expert Consensus Guideline Series: treatment of obsessive-compulsive disorder. Journal Clinical Psychiatry 57(suppl 4):1–72, 1997

18. Alexopoulos GS, Silver JM, Kahn DA, et al (eds): The Expert Consensus Guideline Series: treatment of agitation in older persons with dementia. Postgraduate Medicine Special Report, 1998

19. The Expert Consensus Guideline Series: treatment of posttraumatic stress disorder: the expert consensus panels for PTSD. Journal of Clinical Psychiatry 60(suppl 16):3–76, 1999

20. Canadian clinical practice guidelines for the treatment of schizophrenia. Canadian Journal of Psychiatry 43(suppl 2):25S–40S, 1998

21. Practice parameters for the assessment and treatment of children and adolescents with schizophrenia. Journal of the American Academy of Child and Adolescent Psychiatry 33(suppl 5):616–635, 1994

22. Hughes CW, Emslie GJ, Crismon ML, et al: The Texas Children's Medication Algorithm Project: report of the Texas consensus conference panel on medication treatment of childhood major depressive disorder. Journal of the American Academy of Child and Adolescent Psychiatry 38:1442–1454, 1999

23. Miller AL, Dassori A, Ereshefsky L, et al: Recent issues and developments in antipsychotic use. Psychiatric Clinics of North America: Annual Review of Drug Therapy, in press, 2001

24. Kane J, Honigfeld G, Singer J, et al: Clozapine for the treatment-resistant schizophrenic: a double-blind comparison with chlorpromazine. Archives of General Psychiatry 45:789–796, 1997

25. Sharif Z, Raza A, Ratakonda SS: Comparative efficacy of risperidone and clozapine in the treatment of patients with refractory schizophrenia or schizoaffective disorder: a retrospective analysis. Journal of Clinical Psychiatry 61:498–504, 2000

26. Conley RR, Tamminga CA, Kelly DL, et al: Treatment-resistant schizophrenic patients respond to clozapine after olanzapine nonresponse. Biological Psychiatry 46:73–77, 1999

27. Fava M: Management of nonresponse and intolerance: switching strategies. Journal of Clinical Psychiatry 61(suppl 2):10–12, 2000

28. Nelson JC: Augmentation strategies in depression: 2000. Journal of Clinical Psychiatry 61(suppl 2):13–19, 2000

29. Landen M, Bjorling G, Agren H, et al: A randomized, double-blind, placebo-controlled trial of buspirone in combination with an SSRI in patients with treatment-refractory depression. Journal of Clinical Psychiatry 59:664–668, 1998

30. Perez V, Soler J, Puigdemont D, et al: A double-blind randomized, placebo-controlled trial of pindolol augmentation in depressive patients resistant to serotonin reuptake inhibition. Archives of General Psychiatry 56:375–379, 1999

31. Freeman MP, Stoll AL: Mood stabilizer combinations: a review of safety and efficacy. American Journal of Psychiatry 155:12–21, 1998

32. Janicak PG, Davis JM, Gibbons RD, et al: Efficacy of ECT: a meta-analysis. American Journal of Psychiatry 142:297–302, 1985

33. Brady K, Pearlstein T, Asnis GM, et al: Efficacy and safety of sertraline treatment of posttraumatic stress disorder: a randomized controlled trial. JAMA 283:1837–1844, 2000

34. Cowdry RW, Gardner DL: Pharmacotherapy of borderline personality disorder. Archives of General Psychiatry 45:111–119, 1998

35. Coccaro E, Kavoussi RJ: Fluoxetine and impulsive aggressive behavior in personality-disordered subjects. Archives of General Psychiatry 54:1081–1088, 1996

36. Report of the Surgeon General Conference on Children's Mental Health, Feb 2000. Available at www.surgeongeneral.gov/cmh/childreport.htm)

37. Lehman AF, Steinwachs DM: Patterns of usual care for schizophrenia: initial results from the Schizophrenia Patient Outcomes Research Team (PORT) client survey. Schizophrenia Bulletin 24:11–20, 1998

38. Young AS, Sullivan G, Burnam MA, et al: Measuring the quality of outpatient treatment for schizophrenia. Archives of General Psychiatry 55:611–617, 1998

39. Cabana MD, Rand CS, Powe NR, et al: Why don't physicians follow clinical practice guidelines? A framework for improvement. JAMA 282:1458–1465, 1999

40. Toprac MG, Rush AJ, Conner TM, et al: The Texas Medication Algorithm Project patient and family education program: a consumer-guided initiative. Journal of Clinical Psychiatry 61:477–486, 2000

41. Shiffman RN, Freudigman MD, Brant CA, et al: A guideline implementation system using handheld computers for office management of asthma: effects on adherence and patient outcomes. Pediatrics 105:767–773, 2000

42. Bridging Science and Service: A Report by the National Advisory Mental Health Council's Clinical Treatment and Services Research Workgroup. Rockville, Md, National Institute of Mental Health, 1999

Developing Effective Treatments for Posttraumatic Disorders Among People With Severe Mental Illness

Stanley D. Rosenberg, Ph.D.

Kim T. Mueser, Ph.D.

Matthew J. Friedman, M.D., Ph.D.

Paul G. Gorman, Ed.D.

Robert E. Drake, M.D., Ph.D.

Robert M. Vidaver, M.D.

William C. Torrey, M.D.

Mary K. Jankowski, Ph.D.

Objective: The purpose of the study was to examine strategies for developing effective interventions for clients who have both serious mental illness and posttraumatic symptoms. _Methods:_ The authors conducted searches for articles published between 1970 and 2000, using MEDLINE, PsycLIT, and PILOTS. They assessed current practices, interviewed consumers and providers, and examined published and unpublished documents from consumer groups and state mental health authorities. _Results and conclusions:_ Exposure to trauma, particularly violent victimization, is endemic among clients with severe mental illness. Multiple psychiatric and behavioral problems are associated with trauma, but posttraumatic stress disorder (PTSD) is the most common and best-defined consequence of trauma. Mental health consumers and providers have expressed concerns about several trauma-related issues, including possible underdiagnosis of PTSD, misdiagnosis of other psychiatric disorders among trauma survivors, incidents of retraumatization in the mental health treatment system, and inadequate treatment for trauma-related disorders. Despite consensus that trauma and PTSD symptoms should be routinely evaluated, valid assessment techniques are not generally used by mental health care providers. PTSD is often untreated among clients with serious mental illness, or it is treated with untested interventions. It is important that policy makers, service system administrators, and providers recognize the prevalence and impact of trauma in the lives of people with severe mental illness. The development of effective treatments for this population requires a rational, orderly process, beginning with the testing of theoretically grounded interventions in controlled clinical trials.

Dr. Rosenberg, Dr. Mueser, and Dr. Drake are professors of psychiatry, Dr. Torrey is associate professor of psychiatry, and Dr. Jankowski is a postdoctoral fellow at the New Hampshire–Dartmouth Psychiatric Research Center, 2 Whipple Place, Suite 202, Lebanon, New Hampshire 03766 (e-mail, stanley.d.rosenberg@dartmouth.edu). Dr. Friedman is professor of psychiatry at Dartmouth Medical School and director of the National Center for PTSD in White River Junction, Vermont. Dr. Gorman is assistant professor of psychiatry and director of the West Institute at the New Hampshire–Dartmouth Psychiatric Research Center. Dr. Vidaver is professor of psychiatry at Dartmouth Medical School. This article was originally published in the November 2001 issue of Psychiatric Services.

This series has highlighted the importance of implementing evidence-based practices in the treatment of people who have severe mental illness (1,2). Effective, replicable interventions are available in key areas of need: medications prescribed within specific parameters, self-management of illness, assertive community treatment, family psycho-education, supported employment, and the integration of substance abuse and mental health treatments. Often, however, these tested treatments are not provided to clients of the public mental health system (3). At the same time, resources are being deployed toward services for which empirical support is lacking.

In decisions about the investment of scarce resources in the development of newer interventions, problems and outcomes of particular importance to consumers should receive priority, as should outcomes with strong relationships to the primary symptoms and disabilities associated with severe mental illness (1). In this article, we review evidence that suggests that trauma and posttraumatic stress disorder (PTSD) qualify as priority areas on both counts, and we propose a strategy for developing evidence-based treatments.

A traumatic event involves a direct threat of death, severe bodily harm, or psychological injury that the person finds intensely distressing at the time (4). Common examples of trauma are combat exposure and violent victimization, such as rape and assault. Until recently, exposure to trauma was thought to be relatively rare and to be linked to high-risk experiences, such as wartime military service. However, a series of community studies in the 1990s (5–8) provided evidence that trauma exposure was common, even in middle-class populations. Fifty-six percent of adult respondents in a large, representative national sample reported having experienced at least one traumatic event during their lives (9). These studies also confirmed that many forms of victimization, particularly sexual assault, are greatly underreported (10–12). A few small, early studies (13,14) also suggested that trauma was even more common among people who were in treatment for serious psychiatric illness.

As these findings emerged, a number of conferences were convened to consider the issue of trauma and abuse as it related to clients of the public mental health system (15–17). A major theme was that the abuse of women, particularly sexual abuse, had been ignored or misunderstood by mental health care providers, leaving clients without appropriate care. In the worst cases, female clients were subjected to mental health treatments that exacerbated their posttraumatic symptoms, leading to a negative spiral. That is, coercive interventions, such as involuntary hospitalization and the use of restraints, could worsen posttraumatic symptoms, leading to more prolonged and restrictive care.

In 1994 Jennings (18) published an account of her daughter's tragic experiences dealing with untreated sequelae of trauma in the context of having a serious mental illness. She emphasized the importance of recognizing and treating the effects of childhood sexual abuse among clients with severe mental illness to avoid such spirals and to better help survivors deal with and overcome posttraumatic symptoms. Multiple accounts by trauma survivors with serious mental illness have indicated their dissatisfaction with traditional mental health treatments. Consumers have described episodes of retraumatization and exacerbation of

symptoms due to encounters in the treatment system, such as violence by other clients or forcible restraint by male attendants (15,16).

Harris (19) was one of the first clinicians to publish recommendations for modifying services for women with severe mental illness who were also survivors of sexual abuse trauma. She called for more systematic assessment of trauma history; better staff training; modification of standard services to recognize particular safety, control, and boundary issues facing these clients; and coordination of care across multiple presenting symptoms—for example, substance abuse, psychotic disorder, and PTSD.

The early evidential base for the state trauma initiatives was largely anecdotal, and systematic data for determining priorities and solutions either were inadequate or were not considered.

This growing movement drew attention to trauma and helped stimulate research and programs. Several state-level initiatives were launched to respond to the problems of persons with both severe mental illness and a history of abuse and to address several priorities and perspectives. These initiatives had some important commonalities, including an emphasis on sexual victimization of women and a primary focus on childhood sexual

abuse rather than trauma that may have occurred in adulthood (16,17).

Another important thrust was an emphasis on victimization or retraumatization at the hands of providers or the mental health system itself, including events that served as triggers, reevoking memories of trauma. Providers were often seen as insensitive or demeaning in their responses to trauma survivors. Consumers suggested that clinicians needed to be more aware of trauma-related difficulties and that the treatment system should develop better mechanisms to ensure that trauma survivors receive humane treatment and that their personal rights are respected.

Consumers, advocates, clinicians, and policy makers noted a wide range of trauma-associated problems they wanted to address, including empowerment and recovery; multiple disorders, including acute stress reactions, PTSD, dissociative identity disorder, and disorders of extreme stress not otherwise specified; and general symptoms associated with trauma survivors, such as self-harming behaviors and dissociation. An additional concern was that many clients were misdiagnosed as having major mental illnesses, such as schizophrenia, but were actually trauma survivors with severe or complex PTSD, dissociative identity disorder, and related syndromes.

The concept of trauma-sensitive services was a common component of several state initiatives but had varying definitions. In New York State, emphasis was placed on the identification and acknowledgment of trauma, on recognition of the potential for inadvertent harm to trauma survivors as a result of standard mental health care practices, and on the recovery process of trauma survivors, including the need to enhance their sense of safety and control (17). A Massachusetts Department of Mental Health task force emphasized a specific set of guidelines for assessing clients' history of trauma and to alter restraint and seclusion policies to reduce retraumatization (20). Some consumer-survivors defined trauma-sensitive services more broadly as an antidote to "oppression and injustice within the mental health system" and advocated for more radical reform of the mental health system, with an emphasis on consumer control and challenges to current psychiatric paradigms (21).

The early evidential base for the state trauma initiatives was largely anecdotal, and systematic data for determining priorities and solutions either were inadequate or were not considered in the design of programs. For example, the emphasis on childhood sexual abuse overlooks the most frequent types of trauma reported by people who have severe mental illness (22) and does not consider male clients, who also have high levels of exposure to trauma. In the largest study of trauma exposure among clients with serious mental illness, both men and women were more likely to report having experienced physical abuse than sexual abuse during childhood, and both reported higher overall rates of victimization in adulthood than childhood (unpublished data, Mueser KT, Salyers MP, Rosenberg SD, et al, 2001).

Similarly, data on traumatic events that occur in the treatment setting are scarce. The authors of a recent review were unable to locate published data on either the incidence or the impact on clients of trauma and other harmful events in mental health treatment settings (23). No studies have been published on treatment system modifications that can reduce retraumatization, and rigorous evaluation of such programs would be challenging. Nonetheless, preventing retraumatization of previously abused clients in the mental health treatment system became a major objective of several states (16,20,24).

There is considerable evidence that trauma, abuse, and their effects on people who have serious mental illness are urgent concerns. It is also clear that these issues are highly complex and that the field lacks sufficient information about trauma, PTSD, and effective interventions for this population. Clearer conceptualizations and treatment models—based on sound data—are needed before mental health care providers can implement effective services to address the consequences of trauma. Following recommendations of the National Association of State Mental Health Program Directors (25), we reviewed the available literature on the prevalence, correlates, service use patterns, and assessment issues in relation to trauma exposure and PTSD as well as the published literature on effective interventions for PTSD (26,27).

Methods

For our literature reviews we conducted online searches for articles published between 1970 and 2000 by using MEDLINE, PsycLIT, and PILOTS. Details of these searches can be found in articles by Foa and associates (26,27), Goodman and associates (28), and Mueser and Rosenberg (29). To supplement the literature available through standard online searches, we interviewed consumers and providers and examined published and unpublished documents, from both consumers and state mental health authorities, about current initiatives and recognized needs in relation to trauma and PTSD.

Our consumer informants were a convenience sample of individuals who were active in the recovery movement in New Hampshire and Vermont and consumers and family members who had published in the area of trauma and serious mental illness. Reports of state mental health authorities were obtained only from the eight states that were represented at the National Think Tank hosted by South Carolina in 2000—Connecticut, Maine, Massachusetts, Missouri, New Hampshire, Oregon, South Carolina, and Vermont (30). These states are probably not an unbiased sample of the states as a whole.

Results

Trauma exposure and correlates

People with severe mental illness have a markedly elevated risk of exposure to trauma. About 90 percent of clients with severe mental illness have been exposed to trauma, and most have had multiple exposures (22). Between 34 and 53 percent of clients with severe mental illness report childhood sexual or physical abuse (14,31–33), and 43 to 81 percent report having experienced some type of victimization during their life (13, 34–37). Episodically homeless women with severe mental illness report rates of victimization of 77 to 97 percent (38,39).

Many psychiatric and behavioral difficulties are correlated with trauma exposure in the general population, although specific causal links are not clear. For example, exposure to trauma has been correlated with depression, substance use disorders, eating disorders, personality disorders, chronic pain, somatization, greater use of medical and mental health services, and noncompliance with treatment (40–49).

The correlates of violent victimization among clients with severe mental illness appear to be multifaceted and to affect both the severity of preexisting psychiatric symptoms and clients' use of acute mental health care services. Trauma exposure in psychiatric populations is related to more severe symptoms, such as hallucinations and delusions, depression, suicidality, anxiety, hostility, and dissociation (50–53). Exposure to interpersonal violence is also correlated with more frequent hospitalizations, more time in the hospital, more visits to the emergency department, and nonadherence to treatment (34,50,54,55).

PTSD and correlates

In community studies, PTSD is the most common psychiatric disorder related to trauma exposure and is characterized by three symptom clusters: reexperiencing, avoidance, and hyperarousal (4). About 25 percent of persons who are exposed to trauma develop PTSD, and the disorder is often chronic. The risk of PTSD is related to both the amount and the type of exposure. Recent estimates of the lifetime prevalence of PTSD in the U.S. population range from 8 percent to 12 percent (5,8,9), and the point prevalence is about 2 percent (2.7 percent for women and 1.2 percent for men) (56,57).

People with severe mental illness have high rates of trauma exposure generally and have particularly elevated exposure to the specific types of trauma that carry the highest risk of PTSD—for example, childhood abuse and sexual assault (58–63). Multiple studies of PTSD in this population suggest that current rates of PTSD are in the range of 29 to 43 percent, far in excess of the rates reported in community studies (20,21,51,64–66). Interpretation of these results may be complicated by psychometric issues, particularly symptom overlap. That is, psychotic symptoms have been reported among clients who have a primary diagnosis of PTSD (67), and symptoms of schizophrenia may be confused with or contribute to symptoms of PTSD—for example, hallucinations may be confused with flashbacks, and negative symptoms of schizophrenia may be confused with avoidant symptoms of PTSD (68).

However, there is evidence that PTSD can be diagnosed reliably among clients who have severe mental illness. Although determining the validity of a diagnosis of PTSD is more complex, it has been shown that the severity of PTSD symptoms among clients who have severe mental illness is related to the severity of trauma exposure, as it is in community samples (22,64). It is also possible that persons with severe mental illness have an elevated risk of developing PTSD if they are exposed to a traumatic event. PTSD, like exposure to trauma, is related to worse functioning among clients who are severely mentally ill, including more severe psychiatric symptoms, worse health, and higher rates of psychiatric and medical hospitalization (66).

Effective treatments for PTSD

A growing body of evidence shows that well-delineated, theoretically based interventions are effective in the treatment of PTSD. However, there is little evidence to support the effectiveness of any treatment for the broader set of trauma-related difficulties we have summarized—for example, depression, personality disorders, and substance use disorders (26). In addition, non-PTSD trauma-related disorders are diffuse, vary from one person to another, and have less clear relationships to traumatic events, making measurement more difficult and less reliable. For these reasons we have concluded that developing effective treatments for PTSD per se should be a high priority in the development of trauma services for people with severe mental illness.

Evidence-based treatment guidelines for PTSD are available (26,27). Multiple controlled trials have shown that the most effective interventions for PTSD are those based on cognitive-behavioral therapy approaches, including exposure therapy and cognitive restructuring (26,69). Exposure therapy helps clients decrease avoidance of trauma-related stimuli by encouraging them to confront feared thoughts, feelings, and memories. However, none of the controlled studies of exposure therapy included clients with current, active psychotic illness. Exposure therapy may be limited by high dropout rates (70) and could precipitate relapses of symptoms among vulnerable clients.

Cognitive restructuring, on the other hand, is well tolerated and has been used successfully in trials involving the treatment of other symptoms, such as delusions, with severely mentally ill clients. Cognitive restructuring for PTSD is aimed at helping clients identify distorted or self-defeating thoughts that are often related to traumatic experiences, such as "no one can be trusted"; evaluating whether evidence supports these beliefs; and, if not, altering the beliefs accordingly. More-

> *Psychotic symptoms have been reported among clients who have a primary diagnosis of PTSD, and symptoms of schizophrenia may be confused with or contribute to symptoms of PTSD.*

over, cognitive restructuring has been proved effective for clients who have experienced a variety of types of trauma and clients who met criteria for other disorders, such as alcohol abuse and depression (71).

Evidence for the effectiveness of pharmacotherapy for PTSD is mixed. A few controlled trials have shown significant effects for monoamine oxidase inhibitors (MAOIs) or selective serotonin reuptake inhibitors (SSRIs) in alleviating PTSD symptoms. In the largest studies, effect sizes were modest. The most comprehensive review noted that "dramatic responses to medication have been the exception rather than the rule. MAOIs and SSRIs have been more successful than other drugs" (72). Other PTSD treatments, such as inpatient treatment, psychological debriefing, and group therapy, were judged not to be well supported by research.

Assessment and treatment

Many providers and researchers have been concerned that persons with serious mental illness, whose psychotic distortions or delusions may involve themes of sexual or physical abuse (73), may be unable to provide reliable and valid responses to questions about trauma. Caution is also needed in differentiating symptoms of PTSD from those of clients' primary or co-existing psychiatric disorder. However, several recent studies have shown that trauma exposure and PTSD among clients who have serious mental illness can be reliably assessed with standard instruments (65,74,75).

A study currently under way is investigating the use of computer-assisted interviewing to enhance disclosure and to standardize assessment of trauma and screening for PTSD in this population. Results for more than 150 clients suggest that inpatients receiving acute care as well as outpatients with serious mental illness can respond to assessments of trauma and PTSD reliably and without psychotic distortions that would invalidate their responses (unpublished data, Wolford GL, Rosenberg SD, 2001).

Mueser and Rosenberg (29) also conducted a computerized search of the literature from the past 31 years on PTSD treatment for people with severe mental illness, including the currently used techniques for treating PTSD: psychoeducation, stress management and relaxation, cognitive restructuring, exposure-based treatments, supportive interventions, skills training, pharmacologic treatment, and interpersonal or psychodynamic psychotherapy. Their search located four single-case studies and six open trials but no randomized clinical trials of PTSD interventions for people with possible severe mental illness (76–83).

The open trials were generally reported without quantitative pre-post measures, and none met recommended criteria for treatment outcome studies of PTSD (84)—that is, specified target symptoms, reliable outcome measures, clear inclusion and exclusion criteria, and manual-based, replicable treatment programs. Targeted treatment outcomes were variable and included PTSD symptoms, multiple symptoms associated with adult survivors of childhood sexual abuse, and problems associated with homelessness, substance abuse, poverty, domestic abuse, and mental illness.

Participating clients appeared to be diagnostically heterogeneous, and no data were reported on differential response. Almost no males participated in these trials, and it is not clear whether survivors of nonsexual abuse, such as physical assault, were included. Also, most of the interventions described were multifaceted and complex, and the degree to which they could be adapted to a manual, assessed for model fidelity, or exported to other service settings was unclear.

Two single-case design studies of cognitive-behavioral therapy for women with severe mental illness and PTSD showed improvement in symptoms of PTSD and in psychotic and affective symptoms after treatment (78,79). Contrary to concerns expressed in the literature (85), both of these clients were able to tolerate the PTSD intervention and experienced no other exacerbation of symptoms. If we use standard criteria for determining empirically supported treatments (86), few conclusions about efficacious trauma treatments for people with serious mental illness can be drawn from this review.

However, some consensus about potentially useful interventions can be inferred from these few published studies. First, extensive literature reviews did not locate a single published report that provided evidence that addressing the correlates or sequelae of trauma among persons with severe mental illness, including PTSD, was unsafe or clinically harmful. Second, even critics of state trauma initiatives (87) argue for the use of well-defined, evidence-based interventions for seriously mentally ill clients with posttraumatic symptoms.

Third, trauma treatments for clients with serious mental illness should take place in a context of comprehensive services, such as case

Studies have shown that trauma exposure and PTSD among clients who have serious mental illness can be reliably assessed with standard instruments.

management, medication management, and integrated dual diagnosis treatment when substance abuse problems are present (77,88,89). Finally, the clinical reports in the literature support the hypothesis that trauma interventions are feasible, even in the context of acute or chronic psychotic illness and comorbid substance use disorders (80–82,90).

A number of investigators are currently attempting to develop and evaluate effective treatments for people with serious mental illness who also exhibit posttraumatic symptoms. Two basic types of approaches are used. The first derives from established community mental health interventions and targets adjustment broadly; the second adopts established PTSD interventions for this population and targets PTSD symptoms specifically. In the best-known example of the first type, Harris (89) has developed a multipronged approach for female survivors of trauma who have severe mental illness—the trauma recovery and empowerment model.

The trauma recovery and empowerment model adds a 33-week group intervention to a comprehensive community support and case management approach. Clients are provided with psychoeducation and are taught reframing and problem-solving skills. In the middle stages of the intervention, clients are helped to address trauma experiences more directly, to experience validation from others, and to develop greater self-trust and a greater sense of competence. This intervention is undergoing quasi-experimental evaluation in the Substance Abuse and Mental Health Services Administration Cooperative, a multisite study of women and violence. Fallot and Harris (91) have developed a separate treatment manual for men. The trauma recovery and empowerment model is directed at the broad range of trauma sequelae and does not specifically address PTSD.

As for the second type of intervention, several established PTSD interventions for persons with severe mental illness are being adapted (92–94). These interventions include a three-session psychoeducational intervention, a 12- to 16-session individual cognitive-behavioral treatment, and a 21-session cognitive-behavioral group treatment. The psychoeducational intervention is based on videotapes about trauma and PTSD. The cognitive-behavioral interventions are adapted directly from standard protocols for female survivors of childhood sexual abuse (95) by eliminating the exposure-based elements of treatment and adapting the cognitive restructuring elements (96).

Current trauma services and policy issues

What, then, are public-sector mental health providers doing in this vacuum of empirical data on effective treatments? Because there are no published surveys of current provider practices, this summary is based on reports and other documents from state mental health authorities and on interviews with administrators and providers. Unfortunately, this information is fragmentary and is related primarily to the eight states that reported at the National Association of State Mental Health Program Directors' Think Tank on statewide initiatives that address trauma and PTSD in mental health departments. To the extent that the participants were representative, it appears that service development is in a very early stage. A number of providers have innovated treatments for women that address issues associated with sexual abuse trauma but have not yet subjected these interventions to systematic evaluation. Overall, there is little evidence that empirically based practices are being instituted in routine mental health service settings or even that interventions are being systematically benchmarked in a way that can guide future implementation.

Although a number of state mental health authorities have called for uniform assessment of trauma exposure (24,97), the procedures and methods used to gather these data have often lacked specification and uniformity, and no effort to assess their reliability and validity has been documented. Providers do not appear to have adopted research-based procedures or instruments for screening and assessment. Some states have asked providers to rate clients' history of abuse, but it appears that standardized, reliable techniques are not being used to elicit such a history (20,98).

It is clear from the proceedings of the National Think Tank and interviews with providers and system administrators that consumer demand and providers' concerns are driving efforts to treat the sequelae of trauma among clients with severe mental illness in the absence of data on what constitutes effective treatment. Inpatient and outpatient treatments—in both individual and group formats and with a variety of treatment goals—are being offered to trauma survivors from multiple diagnostic groups. New York State, which has been a leader in

this area, has collated the reports of trauma work groups established in 1995 at each state mental health facility in the *Resource Book on Trauma Assessment and Treatment* (99).

In addition, some states are beginning to train providers in a variety of PTSD treatment models, including the "seeking safety" group approach, which has shown efficacy in a small trial involving women with substance use problems and PTSD (100). The trauma recovery and empowerment model (89) is being introduced or adapted by several states. It appears

Consumer demand and providers' concerns are driving efforts to treat the sequelae of trauma among clients with severe mental illness in the absence of data on what constitutes effective treatment.

that women with a history of childhood sexual abuse are often the primary consumers of these treatments.

Numerous authors (77,101–104), national conferences (15), state mental health authorities (16,17,97–99), the National Association of State Mental Health Program Directors (25), and consumer groups (17) have made recommendations similar to those of the participants in the National Think Tank. All agree on the need for evidence-based clinical guidelines for the assessment and treatment of clients who have a histo-

ry of abuse and trauma (103,104). Most also argue for the rapid implementation of trauma services. The problem, of course, is that it is impossible to deploy evidence-based treatments when there is no evidence base. Moreover, premature policy decisions often have undesirable unintended consequences.

One danger is that providers may feel pressure to try unproven interventions that could be ineffective and could even exacerbate symptoms. Another potential problem is that the resources spent on deployment of these interventions may be needed for other evidence-based services that are inadequately funded. In addition, providers may become invested in standard practices and resist change, even when such a practice is shown to be ineffective and an effective practice becomes available.

Discussion

There is consensus that the field needs to develop effective interventions for people who have severe mental illness and a history of trauma. This situation is analogous to other areas in which effective interventions are lacking. A clear clinical need exists; consumers are demanding these services, and clinicians and mental health administrators are interested in providing them. And although several treatment approaches are available, no empirical evidence of effectiveness is available. There is some urgency to this problem. Clients have a legitimate need for services; providers feel pressure to offer trauma interventions, even in nonstandardized and untested forms; and policy makers feel compelled to establish policies.

Developing effective treatments as rapidly and efficiently as possible requires an orderly, rational process involving contributions from researchers, administrators, providers, and consumers. As we have mentioned, several investigators are conducting pilot studies of interventions adapted from the field of severe mental illness or the field of trauma and PTSD. Both are valid approaches. Small pre-post studies should be conducted to show the feasibility, safety, and potential benefits of treatments and to identify the most appropriate clients for participation. These interventions must also have a reasonable cost and must fit well with current community-based services. Standardized procedures for delivering and measuring the interventions—for example, manuals and fidelity measures—are also needed before clinical trials are conducted.

In proceeding from pilot studies to controlled trials, researchers often prefer to conduct well-designed experiments under carefully controlled conditions—for example, using highly trained clinicians in a university setting with diagnostically homogeneous and uncomplicated patients. They then proceed to studies that use frontline clinicians, routine settings, and more typical community mental health patients. This approach can be useful in many situations, particularly when the intervention needs a great deal of refinement before it can be tested in routine mental health settings. However, this approach does impose the requirement of an extra step before an intervention is ready for broad dissemination, delaying the availability of an effective treatment by at least several years. In addition, some interventions that have been developed in this way have proved too complicated for general adoption or have required resources that are not available at many treatment settings, limiting the impact on routine mental health care.

Thus, to ensure ecological validity, there are advantages to developing and testing psychiatric rehabilitation interventions in the context of standard practice settings. That is, useful interventions must be learned and delivered by a large variety of clinicians and designed to fit into routine mental health programs and settings to apply to the more usual community mental health clients, who often have comorbid disorders and multiple psychosocial problems. These issues can be assessed only through controlled clinical trials under conditions of routine care. Once evidence-based treatments are documented, the final piece of evidence would come from more widespread implementation showing that outcomes can be improved in a large system of care.

Conclusions

It is important that policy makers, service system administrators, and providers recognize the prevalence and impact of trauma in the lives of people who have severe mental illness. In many states, this issue has begun to receive attention, but the treatments offered have not been evidence based and have not been implemented in a way that will lead to cumulative learning for the field. Improving services for clients who have both severe mental illness and PTSD will require the collaboration of consumers, providers, policy makers, and researchers in systematically developing and testing effective treatments that can be broadly disseminated to providers of mental health services. We strongly urge policy makers to support a diversity of approaches and research on effective treatments rather than prematurely establishing policies that are likely to have unintended consequences. ♦

References

1. Drake RE, Goldman HH, Leff HS, et al: Implementing evidence-based practices in routine mental health service settings. Psychiatric Services 52:179–182, 2001

2. Torrey WC, Drake RE, Dixon L, et al: Implementing evidence-based practices for persons with severe mental illness. Psychiatric Services 52:45–50, 2001

3. US Public Health Service: Mental Health: A Report of the Surgeon General. Washington, DC, Department of Health and Human Services, 2000

4. Diagnostic and Statistical Manual of Mental Disorders, 4th ed. Washington, DC, American Psychiatric Association, 1994

5. Breslau N, Davis GC, Andreski P, et al: Traumatic events and posttraumatic stress disorder in an urban population of young adults. Archives of General Psychiatry 48: 216–222, 1991

6. Breslau N, Davis GC, Andreski P: Risk factors for PTSD-related traumatic events: a prospective analysis. American Journal of Psychiatry 152:529–535, 1995

7. Norris F: Epidemiology of trauma: frequency and impact of different potentially traumatic events on different demographic groups. Journal of Consulting and Clinical Psychology 60.409–418, 1992

8. Resnick HS, Kilpatrick DG, Dansky BS, et al: Prevalence of civilian trauma and posttraumatic stress disorder in a representative national sample of women. Journal of Consulting and Clinical Psychology 61: 984–991, 1993

9. Kessler RC, Sonnega A, Bromet E, et al: Posttraumatic stress disorder in the national comorbidity survey. Archives of General Psychiatry 52:1048–1060, 1995

10. Koss MP: Violence against women. American Psychologist 45:374–380, 1990

11. Briere J, Conte JR: Self-reported amnesia for abuse in adults molested as children. Journal of Traumatic Stress 6:2212–2231, 1993

12. Feldhaus KM, Houry D, Kaminsky R: Lifetime sexual assault prevalence rates and reporting practices in an emergency department. Annals of Emergency Medicine 36:23–27, 2000

13. Hutchings PS, Dutton MA: Sexual assault history in a community mental health center clinical population. Community Mental Health Journal 29:59–63, 1993

14. Rose SM, Peabody CG, Stratigeas B: Undetected abuse among intensive case management clients. Hospital and Community Psychiatry 42:499–503, 1991

15. Dare to Vision: Shaping the National Agenda for Women, Abuse, and Mental Health Services. Proceedings of a conference. Arlington, Va, Center for Mental Health Services and Human Resource Association of the Northeast, July 1995

16. Jennings AF, Ralph RO: In Their Own Words: Trauma Advisory Groups Report. Augusta, Me, Maine Department of Mental Health, Mental Health Retardation, and Substance Abuse Services, 1997

17. Mental Health Association in New York State and New York State Office of Mental Health: Proceedings From the Forum on Individuals Diagnosed With Serious Mental Illness Who Are Sexual Abuse Survivors. Albany, New York State Office of Mental Health, 1995

18. Jennings AF: On being invisible in the mental health system. Journal of Mental Health Administration 21:374–387, 1994

19. Harris M: Modifications in service delivery and clinical treatment for women diagnosed with severe mental illness who are also the survivors of sexual abuse trauma. Journal of Mental Health Administration 21:397–406, 1994

20. Task Force on the Restraint and Seclusion of Persons Who Have Been Physically and Sexually Abused: Report and Recommendations. Boston, Massachusetts Department of Mental Health, 1996

21. Deegan PE: Before we dare to vision, we must be willing to see. Keynote address, Dare to Vision: Shaping the National Agenda for Women, Abuse, and Mental Health Services. Proceedings of a conference. Arlington, Va, Center for Mental Health Services and Human Resource Association of the Northeast, July 1995

22. Mueser KT, Goodman LA, Trumbetta SL, et al: Trauma and posttraumatic stress disorder in severe mental illness. Journal of Consulting and Clinical Psychology 66: 493–499, 1998

23. Frueh BC, Dalton ME, Johnson MR, et al: Trauma within the psychiatric setting: con-

ceptual framework, research directions, and policy implications. Administration and Policy in Mental Health 28:147–154, 2000

24. Tucker WH: Clinical issues. OMH Quarterly, Mar 1998, page 3 (published by the New York State Office of Mental Health)

25. Responding to the Behavioral Healthcare Issues of Persons With Histories of Physical and Sexual Abuse: Executive Summary. Alexandria, Va, National Association of State Mental Health Program Directors, 1998

26. Foa EB, Keane TM, Friedman MJ: Guidelines for treatment of PTSD. Journal of Traumatic Stress 13:539–555, 2000

27. Foa EB, Keane TM, Friedman MJ: Effective Treatments for PTSD. New York, Guilford, 2000

28. Goodman LA, Rosenberg SD, Mueser KT, et al: Physical and sexual assault history in women with serious mental illness: prevalence, impact, treatment, and future directions. Schizophrenia Bulletin 23:685–696, 1997

29. Mueser KT, Rosenberg SD: Treatment of PTSD, in Core Approaches for the Treatment of PTSD. Edited by Wilson JP, Friedman MJ, Lindy JD. New York, Guilford, in press

30. Frueh C, Cusack KJ, Hiers TG, et al: Improving public mental health services for trauma victims in South Carolina. Psychiatric Services 52:812–814, 2001

31. Greenfield SF, Strakowski SM, Tohen M, et al: Childhood abuse in first-episode psychosis. British Journal of Psychiatry 164:831–834, 1994

32. Jacobson A, Herald C: The relevance of childhood sexual abuse to adult psychiatric inpatient care. Hospital and Community Psychiatry 41:154–158, 1990

33. Ross CA, Anderson G, Clark P: Childhood abuse and the positive symptoms of schizophrenia. Hospital and Community Psychiatry 45:489–491, 1994

34. Carmen E, Rieker PP, Mills T: Victims of violence and psychiatric illness. American Journal of Psychiatry 141:378–383, 1984

35. Jacobson A: Physical and sexual assault histories among psychiatric outpatients. American Journal of Psychiatry 146:755–758, 1989

36. Jacobson A, Richardson B: Assault experiences of 100 psychiatric inpatients: evidence of the need for routine inquiry. American Journal of Psychiatry 144:508–513, 1987

37. Lipschitz DS, Kaplan ML, Sorkenn JB, et al: Prevalence and characteristics of physical and sexual abuse among psychiatric outpatients. Psychiatric Services 47:189–191, 1996

38. Davies-Netzley S, Hurlburt MS, Hough R: Childhood abuse as a precursor to homelessness for homeless women with severe mental illness. Violence and Victims 11:129–142, 1996

39. Goodman LA, Dutton MA, Harris M: Physical and sexual assault prevalence among episodically homeless women with serious mental illness. American Journal of Orthopsychiatry 65:468–478, 1995

40. Beitchman JH, Zucker KJ, Hood JE, et al: A review of the long term effects of child sexual abuse. Child Abuse and Neglect 16:101–118, 1992

41. Drossman DA, Leserman J, Nachman G, et al: Sexual and physical abuse in women with functional or organic gastrointestinal disorders. Annals of Internal Medicine 113:828–833, 1990

42. Freedy JR, Resnick HS, Kilpatrick DG, et al: The psychological adjustment of recent crime victims in the criminal justice system. Journal of Interpersonal Violence 9:450–468, 1994

43. Golding JM, Stein JA, Siegel JM, et al: Sexual assault history and use of health and mental health services. American Journal of Community Psychology 16:625–643, 1988

44. Moeller TP, Bachman GA, Moeller JR: The combined effects of physical, sexual, and emotional abuse during childhood: long-term health consequences for women. Child Abuse and Neglect 17:623–640, 1993

45. Palmer JA, Palmer LK, Williamson D, et al: Childhood abuse as a factor in attrition from drug rehabilitation. Psychological Reports 76:879–882, 1995

46. Polusny MA, Follette VM: Long-term correlates of child sexual abuse: theory and review of the empirical literature. Applied and Preventive Psychology 4:143–166, 1995

47. Rapkin AJ, Kames LD, Darke LL, et al: History of physical and sexual abuse in women with chronic pelvic pain. Obstetrics and Gynecology 76:92, 1990

48. Rosenberg HJ, Rosenberg SD, Williamson PJ, et al: A comparative study of trauma and PTSD prevalence in epileptic and psychogenic non-epileptic seizure patients. Epilepsia 41:447–452, 2000

49. Rosenberg HJ, Rosenberg SD, Wolford GL, et al: The relationship between trauma, PTSD, and medical utilization in three high-risk medical populations. Psychiatry in Medicine 30:247–259, 2000

50. Briere J, Woo, R, McRae B, et al: Lifetime victimization history, demographics, and clinical status in female psychiatric emergency room patients. Journal of Nervous and Mental Disease 185:95–101, 1997

51. Craine LS, Henson CE, Colliver JA, et al: Prevalence of a history of sexual abuse among female psychiatric patients in a state hospital system. Hospital and Community Psychiatry 39:300–304, 1988

52. Figueroa EF, Silk KR, Huth A, et al: History of childhood sexual abuse and general psychopathology. Comprehensive Psychiatry 38:23–30, 1997

53. Goodman LA, Dutton MA, Harris M: The relationship between violence dimensions and symptom severity among homeless, mentally ill women. Journal of Traumatic Stress 10:51–70, 1997

54. Goodman LA, Salyers MP, Mueser KT, et al: Recent victimization in women and men with severe mental illness: prevalence and correlates. Journal of Traumatic Stress, in press

55. Vidaver RM, Salyers MP, Mueser KT, et al: Impact of recent victimization on course of illness and service utilization in persons with severe mental illness. Presented at the annual meeting of the American Psychiatric Association, Chicago, May 13–18, 2000

56. Perkonigg A, Kessler RC, Storz S, et al: Traumatic events and post-traumatic stress disorder in the community: prevalence, risk factors, and comorbidity. Acta Psychiatrica Scandinavica 101:46–59, 2000

57. Stein MB, Walker JR, Hazen AL, et al: Full and partial posttraumatic stress disorder: findings from a community survey. American Journal of Psychiatry 154:1114–1119, 1997

58. Davidson J, Smith R: Traumatic experiences in psychiatric outpatients. Journal of Traumatic Stress 3:459–475, 1990

59. O'Neill K, Gupta K: Post-traumatic stress disorder in women who were victims of childhood sexual abuse. Irish Journal of Psychological Medicine 8:124–127, 1991

60. Resnick HS, Kilpatrick DG, Dansky BS, et al: Prevalence of civilian trauma and post-traumatic stress disorder in a representative national sample of women. Journal of Consulting and Clinical Psychology 61:984–991, 1993

61. Rothbaum BO, Foa EB, Riggs D, et al: A prospective examination of post-traumatic stress disorder in rape victims. Journal of Traumatic Stress 5:455–475, 1992

62. Breslau N, Kessler RC, Chilcoat HD, et al: Trauma and post-traumatic stress disorder in the community: the 1996 Detroit area survey of trauma. American Journal of Psychiatry 55:626–632, 1998

63. Halligan SL, Yehuda R: Risk factors for PTSD. PTSD Quarterly 11(3):1–8, 2000

64. Cascardi M, Mueser KT, DeGirolomo J, et al: Physical aggression against psychiatric inpatients by family members and partners: a descriptive study. Psychiatric Services 47:531–533, 1996

65. Mueser KT, Salyers MP, Rosenberg SD, et al: A psychometric evaluation of trauma and PTSD assessments in persons with severe mental illness. Psychological Assessment 13(1):110–117, 2001

66. Switzer GE, Dew MA, Thompson K, et al: Posttraumatic stress disorder and service utilization among urban mental health center clients. Journal of Traumatic Stress 12:25–39, 1999

67. Lindley SE, Carlson E, Sheikh J: Psychotic symptoms in posttraumatic stress disorder. CNS Spectrums 5(9):52–57, 2000

68. Rosenberg SD, Mueser KT, Fox MB: Issues in the dual diagnosis of schizophrenia and PTSD: reliability and validity. Present-

ed at Congress on Associated Psychiatric Syndromes in Schizophrenia, Chicago, May 14–18, 2000

69. Solomon JD: Psychosocial treatment of posttraumatic stress disorder. Session: Psychotherapy in Practice 3(4):27–41, 1997

70. Foy DW, Kagan BL, McDermott C, et al: Practical parameters in the use of flooding for treating chronic PTSD. Clinical Psychology and Psychotherapy 3(3):169–175, 1996

71. Tarrier N, Pilgrim H, Sommerfield C, et al: Cognitive and exposure therapy in the treatment of PTSD. Journal of Consulting and Clinical Psychology 67:13–18, 1999

72. Friedman MJ, Davidson JRT, Mellman TA, et al: Pharmacotherapy, in Effective Treatments for PTSD. Edited by Foa EB, Keane TM, Friedman MJ. New York, Guilford, 2000

73. Coverdale JH, Grunebaum H: Sexuality and family planning, in Handbook of Social Functioning in Schizophrenia. Edited by Mueser KT, Tarrier N. Boston, Allyn and Bacon, 1998

74. Meyer IH, Munzenmaier K, Cancienne J, et al: Reliability and validity of a measure of sexual and physical abuse histories among women with serious mental illness. Child Abuse and Neglect 20:213–219, 1996

75. Goodman LA, Thompson KM, Weinfurt K, et al: Reliability of reports of violent victimization and PTSD among men and women with SMI. Journal of Traumatic Stress 12:587–599, 1999

76. Harris M: Treating sexual abuse trauma with dually diagnosed women. Community Mental Health Journal 32:371–385, 1996

77. Alexander MJ, Muenzenmaier K: Trauma, addiction, and recovery: addressing public health: epidemics among women with severe mental illness, in Women's Mental Health Services: A Public Health Perspective. Edited by Levin B, Lubotsky B, Andrea K. Thousand Oaks, Calif, Sage, 1998

78. Mueser KT, Taylor KL: A cognitive-behavioral approach, in Sexual Abuse in the Lives of Women Diagnosed With Severe Mental Illness. Edited by Harris M, Landis CL. Amsterdam, Harwood, 1997

79. Nishith P, Hearst DE, Mueser KT, et al: PTSD and major depression: methodological and treatment considerations in a single case design. Behavior Therapy 26:319–335, 1995

80. Herder DD, Redner L: The treatment of childhood sexual trauma in chronically mentally ill adults. Health and Social Work 16:50–57, 1991

81. Stowe H, Harris M: A social skills approach to trauma recovery for women diagnosed with serious mental illness, in Sexual Abuse in the Lives of Women Diagnosed With Severe Mental Illness. Edited by Harris M, Landis CL. Amsterdam, Harwood, 1997

82. Talbot NL, Houghtalen RP, Cyrulik S, et al: Women's safety in recovery: group therapy for patients with a history of childhood sexual abuse. Psychiatric Services 49:213–217, 1998

83. Muenzenmaier K, Sampson DE: Understanding and Dealing With Sexual Abuse Trauma: An Educational Group for Women. Albany, New York Office of Mental Health, 1998

84. Foa EB, Meadows EA: Psychosocial treatments for posttraumatic stress disorder: a critical review. Annual Review of Psychology 48:449–480, 1997

85. Solomon SD, Davidson JRT: Trauma: prevalence, impairment, service use, and cost. Journal of Clinical Psychiatry 58(suppl 9):5–11, 1997

86. Chambless DL, Ollenick TH: Empirically supported psychological interventions: controversies and evidence. Annual Review of Psychology 52:685–716, 2001

87. Satel SL: Who needs trauma initiatives? Psychiatric Services 52:815, 2001

88. Harris M, Landis CL (eds): Sexual Abuse in the Lives of Women Diagnosed With Serious Mental Illness. Amsterdam, Harwood, 1997

89. Harris M: The Community Connections Trauma Work Group: Trauma Recovery and Empowerment: A Clinician's Guide for Working With Women in Groups. New York, Free Press, 1998

90. Harris M (ed): Sexual Abuse Trauma Among Women Diagnosed With Severe Mental Illness. Newark, NJ, Gordon and Breach, 1997

91. Fallot RD, Harris M, and the Community Connections Men's Trauma Workgroup: Men's Trauma Recovery and Empowerment Model: A Clinician's Guide to Working With Male Trauma Survivors in Groups. Washington, DC, Community Connections, 2001

92. Descamps MJ, Salyers MP, Jankowski MK, et al: Modification of a Protocol for Treating PTSD in Women with Severe Mental Illness. Presented at the annual meeting of the International Society for Traumatic Stress Studies, Miami, November 14–17, 1999

93. Rosenberg SD: Identification and Treatment of PTSD in People With SMI. Grand rounds presented at New Hampshire Hospital, Concord, November 18, 1999

94. Rosenberg SD, Mueser KT, Friedman MJ: Modified PTSD Treatment for People with Severe Mental Illness. Presented at the Congress of the European Association for Behavioural and Cognitive Therapies, Granada, Spain, September 26–28, 2000

95. Foa EB, Dancu CV, Zayfert C, et al: Therapist Guide: Brief Cognitive Behavior Therapy for Post-Traumatic Stress Disorder in Survivors of Childhood Sexual Abuse. White River Junction, Vt, National Center for PTSD, Veterans Affairs Medical and Regional Office Center, 1997

96. Marks I, Lovell K, Noshirvani H, et al: Treatment of posttraumatic stress disorder by exposure and/or cognitive restructuring. Archives of General Psychiatry 55:317–325, 1998

97. A Five Year Plan for Behavioral Health Services in New Hampshire: 2000–2005. Concord, NH, New Hampshire Division of Behavioral Health, 1999

98. Frueh C, Cousins V, Hiers T, et al: Current status of trauma assessment and treatment in the Department of Mental Health, South Carolina Department of Mental Health. Trauma Initiative Newsletter 1(1):5, 2001

99. Trauma Assessment and Treatment Resource Book. Albany, New York State Office of Mental Health, 1998

100. Najavits LM, Weiss RD, Shaw SR et al: "Seeking safety": outcome of a new cognitive-behavioral psychotherapy for women with posttraumatic stress disorder and substance dependence. Journal of Traumatic Stress 11:437–456, 1998

101. Harris M, Fallot RD: Envisioning a trauma-informed service system: a vital paradigm shift. New Directions for Mental Health Services, no 89:3–22, 2001

102. Auslander MW, Bustin-Baker C, Cousins V, et al: Trauma and abuse histories: connections to diagnoses of mental illness: implications for policy and service delivery. Position paper. National Association of Consumer/Survivor Mental Health Administrators, July 1998

103. Connecticut Trauma Initiative Summary: Draft System of Clinical Trauma Services. Hartford, Connecticut Department of Mental Health and Addiction Services, 2001

104. A Description of Who We Are and What We Do. Augusta, Maine Department of Mental Health, Mental Retardation, and Substance Abuse Services, 2000

Evidence-Based Practice in Child and Adolescent Mental Health Services

Kimberly Hoagwood, Ph.D.
Barbara J. Burns, Ph.D.
Laurel Kiser, Ph.D.
Heather Ringeisen, Ph.D.
Sonja K. Schoenwald, Ph.D.

The authors review the status, strength, and quality of evidence-based practice in child and adolescent mental health services. The definitional criteria that have been applied to the evidence base differ considerably across treatments, and these definitions circumscribe the range, depth, and extensionality of the evidence. The authors describe major dimensions that differentiate evidence-based practices for children from those for adults and summarize the status of the scientific literature on a range of service practices. The readiness of the child and adolescent evidence base for large-scale dissemination should be viewed with healthy skepticism until studies of the fit between empirically based treatments and the context of service delivery have been undertaken. Acceleration of the pace at which evidence-based practices can be more readily disseminated will require new models of development of clinical services that consider the practice setting in which the service is ultimately to be delivered.

As is true with any newly popularized term, the term "evidence-based" has an almost intuitive ring of credibility to it. It brings to mind images of tree-lined and stately buildings fronted with Grecian columns and filled with persons wearing white coats, speaking in hushed tones, and offering reassurances. But this ring may be hollow. As Montaigne noted, "Nothing is so firmly believed as what we least know," and as Valery warned, "That which has been delivered by everyone, always and everywhere, has every chance of being false."

There are as many definitions of what constitutes "evidence" as there are definitions of what constitutes a "service." More important, the use of the term "evidence-based practice" presupposes agreement as to how the evidence was generated, what the evidence means, and how or when the practice can be implemented.

We suggest that before this term becomes a slogan, it may be wise to examine the presuppositions behind it, acknowledge the limitations of what is sometimes characterized as evidence-based practice, and, in the next generation of services research, attend to implementation issues at the front end.

Much of what passes for research on evidence-based practice in the field of child and adolescent mental health might more aptly be described as clinical treatment efficacy research. In this article we first describe how evidence-based practice is being defined in the field of child and adolescent mental health, the characteristics of children and of services that pose special challenges in creating evidence-based practices, and the state of research evidence for treatments and services. Finally, we explain why healthy skepticism about current evidence-based practices is not unreasonable.

Definitional applications

In the field of children's mental health services research, the term "evidence-based practice" refers to a body of scientific knowledge about service practices—for example, referral, assessment, and case management—or about the impact of clinical treatments or services on the mental health problems of children and adolescents. The knowledge base is created through the application of scientific methods that examine the impact of certain practices on outcomes for the child or adolescent and his or her family. Evidence-based practice is a shorthand term that denotes the quality, robustness, or validity of scientific evidence as it is brought to bear on these issues. Although the term can and has been applied to preventive strategies, here we focus on treatments and services for children and adolescents who have been identified as having clinical disorders.

In the child and adolescent mental health services field, the term "evidence-based" is most often used to

Dr. Hoagwood and Dr. Ringeisen are affiliated with the National Institute of Mental Health in Bethesda, Maryland. Dr. Burns is with Duke University in Durham, North Carolina. Dr. Kiser is with the University of Maryland in Baltimore. Dr. Schoenwald is with the Medical University of South Carolina in Charleston. Send correspondence to Dr. Hoagwood at the National Institute of Mental Health, 6001 Executive Boulevard, Bethesda, Maryland 20817 (e-mail, kh32p@nih.gov). This article was originally published in the September 2001 issue of Psychiatric Services.

differentiate therapies—generally psychosocial—that have been studied with varying degrees of rigor from therapies that are used but have not been studied or have not been studied well. For example, Kazdin (1) has described four domains that constitute criteria for assessing an evidence base: a theory to relate a hypothesized mechanism to a clinical problem, basic research to assess the validity of the mechanism, preliminary outcome evidence to show that a therapeutic approach changes the relevant outcomes, and process-outcome connections, which display the relationships between process change and clinical outcomes. In essence, Kazdin has defined a process for attaining a valid and substantiated theory about the impact therapy has on a patient.

Operational criteria were proposed by the division of clinical psychology of the American Psychological Association in 1998 and were applied to studies of specific childhood syndromes (2,3). According to these criteria, treatments are to be supported by either group design or single-subject experiments, and studies should clearly describe characteristics of the subjects. For a treatment to be considered "well established," two or more studies must show that it is superior to medication, placebo, or an alternative treatment or that it is equivalent to an already established treatment, or nine single-subject case studies must be conducted to establish its equivalence or superiority. Well-established treatments have been identified for attention-deficit hyperactivity disorder (ADHD)—for example, behavioral parent training and classroom behavior modification (4); for conduct problems—for example, parent training (5); and for phobias—for example, participant modeling and reinforced practice (6).

For an intervention to be considered "probably efficacious," two or more studies must show it to be superior to a wait-list control condition or one experiment must meet the criteria for a well-established treatment, or three single-case studies must be conducted. Treatments that are probably efficacious have been identified for depression and anxiety disorders—for

example, cognitive-behavioral therapy (6,7)—and ADHD, conduct problems, and phobias. Studies of psychosocial interventions among children and adolescents for autism, anorexia and bulimia, posttraumatic stress disorder, bipolar disorder, obsessive-compulsive disorder, panic disorder, and substance abuse have not yet met the criteria for being considered well-established or probably efficacious.

Another approach to defining the evidence base in child research has arisen from the Interdisciplinary Committee on Evidence-Based Youth Mental Health Care, with formal participation by the American Academy of Pediatrics, the American Academy

---

*Much
of what passes
for research on
evidence-based practice
in the field of child and
adolescent mental health
might more aptly be
described as clinical
treatment efficacy
research.*

---

of Child and Adolescent Psychiatry, and the American Psychological Association's divisions of clinical child psychology and school psychology. This committee has built on the work of the American Psychological Association but has attempted to broaden the system to include psychosocial as well as pharmacologic treatments that are scientifically supported (8).

A manual has been developed for use by reviewers of outcome research to enable coding of studies according to highly specified criteria. For treatments to be classified as evidence

based, at least two between-group design studies with a minimum of 30 subjects must be conducted across studies representing the same age group and receiving the same treatment for the same target problem, at least two within-group or single case design studies with the same parameters must be conducted, or there must be a combination of these. Further, a majority of the applicable studies must support the treatment, and the protocol must show acceptable adherence to the treatment manual.

The ultimate goal is to develop an archive of data from clinical trials for all treatment studies and to periodically update this archive such that it can provide research syntheses and meta-analyses to summarize treatment research for children and adolescents (8). This process is not unlike that proposed by the Cochrane Collaborative Group, which has been the primary standard setter for evidence-based reviews in medicine. The Cochrane Collaborative has formed the foundation for many of the projects for the Agency on Healthcare Research and Quality (9).

Finally, the term "evidence-based" has been used to refer to analytic reviews of bodies of studies on a target problem or program. For example, meta-analytic reviews of psychotherapy treatment studies—which usually meet less stringent criteria than those we have described—have been widely cited as suggestive of the strength of the evidence for these therapies (10–12) and as evidence that psychotherapy treatments are as effective for children as they are for adults (12). In addition, several recent reviews of interventions, such as family preservation and school-based services, have set inclusion criteria—for example, a randomized clinical trial, use of established outcome measures, and use of a comparison group—and then synthesized the strength of the evidence for or against the effectiveness of these types of services (13–16).

From a scientific standpoint, applying the same criteria to studies of pharmacological, psychosocial, or prevention interventions is probably warranted. Scientific justification rests on relatively well-accepted principles of control (17). However, there are important differences among these interventions in the ways in which they do—or do not—have regulatory backing.

In pharmaceutical medicine, evidence-based approaches have been built into the regulatory standards developed by the Food and Drug Administration (FDA) to review scientific evidence and identify effective medications. The strength of the evidence for pharmacologic treatments is regulated by the FDA, and an industry has grown up around this regulation, whereas the strength of the evidence for the effectiveness of psychotherapies and other nonpharmacological interventions lies only in the knowledge base created by researchers.

Pharmaceutical companies cannot distribute or advertise a pharmaceutical agent unless it has been approved by the FDA. The existence of regulatory authority over the distribution of effective—and therefore profitable—therapies does not exist for psychosocial treatments or services. Consequently the incentive system for the growth of these therapies is vastly different and largely academic (18).

Evidence-based practice for children's services

Children's versus adults' services

First, although to be human is to develop (in the French sense of *de-enveloper* or un-envelop), children undergo more rapid physiological, neuronal, and psychological changes over a briefer period than adults. The rapidity of this development implies that for evidence-based practice to be meaningful, it has to take into account developmental conditions that affect the durability of the effects of treatment. An evidence-based practice that is effective in the treatment of adolescent depression may well be ineffective or even harmful for children who have not reached puberty.

Attention to developmental increments in the creation of evidence-based practices for children and adolescents means attention not only to age-related changes but also to the complex and dynamic interactions among the child, the family, and the environmental context that accompany maturation (19). In the field of

child and adolescent mental health, answers to questions about the evidence base for services are not meaningful if developmental issues have been ignored.

Second, the creation of a treatment for a child is rarely undertaken without consideration of the family context. In fact, some have argued that even the notion of what constitutes a mental illness cannot be ascertained without knowledge of the interaction between the child and his or her family (20,21). Beyond this interaction, parental perceptions of the nature of presenting problems differ substan-

> An evidence-based practice that is effective in the treatment of adolescent depression may well be ineffective or even harmful for children who have not reached puberty.

tially from the child's perceptions (22). The nature of the diagnosis itself is contextually bound for children and adolescents to a far greater degree than is true for adults (23). Although involvement of caregivers is important in implementation of evidence-based practices for adults, in child mental health research the family is central not only to the development of the treatment or service but also to the understanding of the diagnosis itself.

Third, evidence-based practices for children differ from those for adults in that the types of services for which an evidence-based practice is developed will necessarily involve substan-

tially different service venues. For example, 70 to 80 percent of the mental health services received by children who have mental health problems are provided by schools (24). The adult analog is likely to be the workplace. Yet an evidence-based practice for treating, say, ADHD in a school setting—for example, classroom management by a teacher—is unlikely to be similar to an evidence-based practice developed for treating inattention in the workplace. Issues related to the context or setting of the service place very different demands on the provider of the treatment and on the recipient.

Because of these contextual differences, a wide range of providers will need to be trained to provide the evidence-based practice. Children who have mental health needs may come to the attention of professionals in schools, primary care offices, welfare systems, or detention facilities. The fragmentation of the mental health service system means that for evidence-based practice to reach those who provide care to children, a range of training curricula, materials, and approaches must be developed and specifically tailored for the providers in these systems.

A short history

Until recently, there has been no evidence to summarize, critique, or review in the field of child and adolescent services. In fact, from a historical standpoint it is interesting that the concept of childhood mental illnesses did not arise until the late 19th century. These illnesses were typically not seen as unique to children or distinguishable from adult mental illnesses until the early part of the 20th century. The first English-language text on child psychiatry was published in 1935 (25). The first serious attempts to assess the use of mental health services by children and adolescents were begun in the late 1980s.

Two factors galvanized developments in children's mental health services: recognition that these services were scattered across a vast array of service organizations and systems, including schools, child welfare agencies, pediatric health settings, and juvenile corrections facilities, and recognition that fewer than 20 percent of children who had identified mental health needs received help (24).

The first development was state-level activities to create coordinated points of entry for delivery of mental health services, organized largely under the auspices of the Child and Adolescent Service System Program. This initiative was given principled footing through the creation of a model for revamping children's services. The system-of-care model, developed by Stroul and Friedman (26), articulated a series of values and principles centered on maintaining children in their communities, coordinating services, involving families centrally in delivery and planning of treatments and services, and instantiating attention to the cultural relevance of services. After these principles were developed, the services included in a continuum of care were delineated.

The second development was the creation of a scientific agenda centered on examining the relationship between children's needs for psychiatric care and the availability of such care. The two major efforts in this direction were the Great Smoky Mountains study (27,28) and the study of methods for the epidemiology of children and adolescents (29,30). Both studies found that 4 to 8 percent of children between the ages of nine and 17 years had severe psychiatric disorders and that only about 20 percent of children with the most serious needs were receiving mental health services (24,27,29,31).

During the mid-1990s, the scientific research agenda redirected attention to the quality of the clinical treatments within service systems. The system-of-care studies by Bickman (32,33) showed that system coordination alone improved access to services for children and families and satisfaction with services and also reduced hospitalization and other restrictive forms of care. However, these studies also showed that clinical outcomes for children—for example, alleviation of symptoms, functioning, or reduction of impairments—were the same whether children were receiving coordinated services through systems of care or were receiving usual services.

As a result of these findings, attention was shifted away from general studies of "systemness" to the clinical effectiveness of services within these systems of care and especially to the types, dosages, and intensity of treatments delivered (34–36). In particular, the transportability of efficacious clinical treatments into mental health service systems was highlighted as a critical research area (37–39). To this end, Burns (40) proposed the creation of a research agenda on clinical interventions for youths that would accomplish four tasks: synthesize, through reviews of the evidence base, the status of science on promising interventions; assess the adequacy of quality indicators to improve standards of clinical practice; evaluate the adequacy of outcome measures; and develop a new research phase model for connecting research to practice. The latter activity was subsequently proposed by Weisz and Weersing (18) as well as by Hoagwood and colleagues (41).

As a result of this new focus on bridging science and policy and strengthening knowledge about the efficacy and effectiveness of mental health services (42), a series of studies has been undertaken by a number of investigators, focusing on questions about the effectiveness of manual-based services for children who have a range of serious psychiatric impairments and the effectiveness of practice strategies for enhancing engagement with services.

Types of practices used

Acceptability of engagement and treatment. Treatments that fail to reach those who stand to benefit from them cannot be said to be effective. Unfortunately, inaccessibility of services and termination of treatment are problems that plague the delivery of mental health care. Among children whose families do seek outpatient mental health treatment, 40 to 60 percent may discontinue services before formal completion of treatment (43). Moreover, these families typically do not use outpatient services for very long. Armbruster and Fallon (44) showed that most children who enter outpatient treatment attend for only one or two sessions. There is also

evidence that children from especially vulnerable populations—children of single mothers, children living in poverty, and children from minority groups—and children who have serious presenting problems are less likely to stay in treatment beyond the first session and more likely to discontinue treatment prematurely (45,46).

However, successful efforts can be made to enhance a family's service engagement and to decrease rates of premature termination of treatment. A variety of studies have been undertaken to identify and reduce barriers to service engagement and to increase the participation of minority families in services by using brief telephone interviews before service entry (47–49).

Empirically supported psychosocial outpatient treatments. Meta-analyses of experimental child psychotherapy intervention trials point to a consistent beneficial effect of treatment compared with no treatment (11,50–52). These effects are comparable to those found for adult psychotherapy (10). A similar analysis that summarized a less extensive literature on the treatment effects of therapies conducted in clinical practice settings, as opposed to research settings, found almost no difference between treatment and no treatment (12). In fact, the effect size was negative, falling well below the effects typically found in experimental studies. Consequently, the evidence suggests that psychosocial interventions for children can successfully reduce symptoms associated with childhood mental disorders when conducted in research-based settings; however, the impact of these therapies in clinical practice settings is only now being studied (18).

Family-focused treatments. Because the family plays a major role in the social and emotional development of children, family-focused interventions have long been a part of child and adolescent mental health treatment. Meta-analysis of family-focused treatments shows the general effectiveness of such treatments (19). Controlled trials indicate the effectiveness of family-based interventions for physical child abuse and neglect; conduct problems, including ADHD;

emotional disturbance, specifically anxiety, depression, and grief; toileting problems; and psychosomatic concerns (20). Effective family-based treatments are typically short-term, are offered on an outpatient basis, and have cognitive-behavioral, structural, or strategic foundations. Frequently they are combined with individual therapies and medication management.

Integrated community-based treatment. One criticism of empirically supported psychosocial interventions is that their focus on specific diagnosable disorders does not adequately take account of the heterogeneity of the psychiatric problems that a majority of children have when they present at mental health clinics (53). A series of studies on integrated service models for children who have multiple co-occurring disorders has been examining a range of service modalities, including intensive case management, treatment foster care, and home-based services.

Studies of clinically oriented, intensive case management have found that children who have specially trained case managers require fewer restrictive services, such as psychiatric hospitalizations, than children who do not (54,55). Similar reductions in the number of inpatient hospitalizations have been found for youths with substance use problems (55). The use of case managers in community-based interdisciplinary treatment teams has also been found to improve standard-practice foster care through reductions in the number of placement changes and the number of runaway episodes among older youths (56). Multiple uncontrolled studies of case management services have been conducted in the context of wraparound care (57). These studies have shown that case management services can improve children's positive adjustment, decrease negative behaviors, and improve the stability of community living environments.

A series of studies have tested the impact of therapeutic foster care services for children who have multiple comorbid mental disorders. In a therapeutic foster care environment, a child is placed in a home with foster parents who have received specialized training to work with children who have emotional or behavioral problems. Results from these studies have shown decreases in aggressive behavior and increases in positive adjustment at the conclusion of placement (56–58). Chamberlain and Reid (59) compared treatment outcomes for youths from a state psychiatric hospital who were placed in either therapeutic foster care or usual community care and found that those in therapeutic foster care had fewer re-institutionalizations and more rapid behavioral improvement. In addition,

---

Seventy to 80 percent of children who receive mental health services receive them in school; for many children the school system provides their only form of mental health treatment.

---

youths in the experimental group had less frequent posttreatment incarcerations and criminal referrals and more frequent placements with parents or relatives in the year after treatment (60). In addition, the costs of this service were significantly lower than those of other residential placements (60).

Finally, home-based service models have been developed for children who have serious emotional disturbances. One rigorously studied home-based intervention is multisystemic therapy, the primary goal of which is to develop independent skills among youths who have behavioral

problems and their parents to cope with family, peer, school, and neighborhood problems through brief (three to four months) and intense (sometimes daily) treatment (61). Treatment strategies integrate empirically based treatment approaches— for example, behavioral training for parents, cognitive-behavioral therapies, and functional family therapy— to address the problems of children and adolescents across environmental contexts.

Eight randomized trials of multisystemic therapy have been conducted, and the results have been among the strongest found for children's services. Among a group of chronic juvenile offenders, those who received multisystemic therapy had lower rates of recidivism and out-of-home placements 59 weeks after treatment and lower arrest rates more than two years after treatment (62). Similar results were found when multisystemic therapy was compared with individual therapy in a different group of juvenile offenders (63).

A recent study comparing multisystemic therapy with emergency psychiatric hospitalization among children and adolescents with serious psychiatric impairments has found that multisystemic therapy can safely reduce rates of psychiatric hospitalization and improve the functioning of youths and their families (64,65). The effects of multisystemic therapy have been further demonstrated among juvenile sex offenders (66) and abused or neglected children (67). Researchers evaluating multisystemic therapy suggest that adequate supervision, training of therapists, and institutional program support are essential to successful outcomes (65).

School-based interventions. Seventy to 80 percent of children who receive mental health services receive them in school; for many children the school system provides their only form of mental health treatment (24). About 45 studies of school-based interventions for children with emotional or behavioral problems, covering a 15-year period, were recently reviewed (15). Among these studies, a range of effective individual, classroom, and targeted interventions were identified.

The empirically supported treatments for childhood behavioral problems that are effective in school settings include targeted classroom-based contingency management for children with a diagnosis of ADHD (4) and children with other conduct problems (5). Contingency management also appears to successfully reduce aggression when implemented across entire classrooms. The "good-behavior game," a classroom-based behavior-management strategy for first-grade students, has demonstrated long-term benefits in reducing disruptive behaviors in middle school (68,69). Behavioral consultation to teachers to help them accommodate difficult students has been found to reduce the number of special-education referrals and placements and to reduce teachers' reports of students' behavioral problems (70).

School-based preventive interventions designed to target children who are at risk of emotional or behavioral problems have also been shown to alleviate symptoms and to increase the use of positive coping strategies. Cognitive group interventions to modify adolescents' depressive thinking styles have been associated with a reduced risk of the development of full depression (71). Similarly, a group intervention to teach social problem-solving skills to elementary school children with elevated depressive symptoms demonstrated reductions in reported depression, even one year after the intervention (72). There is also evidence that school-based preventive interventions reduce the risk of conduct problems. Successful interventions typically involve multiple components that target classroom, home, and peer environments (73).

Psychopharmacology. About 3.5 million child outpatient physician visits a year result in a prescription for a psychotropic medication (74). Furthermore, prescription rates for psychotropic medications for children are increasing, even among very young children (75). Clinical trials of psychotropic medications are needed for many childhood mental disorders. Despite the widespread use of these medications, surprisingly few randomized controlled studies have been conducted (16). Many medication choices and algorithms continue to be based on the experience of the individual practitioner or on standards of care for adults, with some notable exceptions (76).

In addition, proper medication selection is only one factor in successful pharmacologic treatment. The recent National Institute of Mental Health multimodal treatment study of ADHD found that clinical outcomes for participants who received careful medication management, including systematic titration to the optimal dosage, were superior to clinical outcomes associated with routine prescription of the same medication delivered in the usual manner in the

Many medication choices and algorithms continue to be based on the experience of the individual practitioner or on standards of care for adults, with some notable exceptions.

community (77). The differences in outcomes seem to have been a result of management practices associated with participation in the medication treatment group.

Weisz and Jensen (16) recently reviewed evidence of the efficacy of child pharmacotherapy by using criteria established for the International Psychopharmacology Algorithm Project (78). According to these criteria, a drug is considered efficacious if its equivalency or superiority have been demonstrated through random-assignment, control group comparison

and the results are replicated in one or more similarly well-controlled studies. In addition, the National Institute of Mental Health recently commissioned six scientific reviews of published studies of the safety and efficacy of psychotropic medications for children (79): psychostimulants (80), mood stabilizers and antimanic agents (81), selective serotonin reuptake inhibitors (SSRIs) (82), tricyclic antidepressants (83), antipsychotic agents (84), and miscellaneous agents (85). These reviews identified several psychotropic medications for which there is empirical support for use in both externalizing and internalizing disorders in childhood, most prominent among which are psychostimulants for children with ADHD.

For depression, the most commonly studied pharmacologic agents have been the tricyclic antidepressants, but they have not been shown to be effective in treating childhood depression. Newer and safer agents, such as SSRIs, are being studied more frequently in the treatment of childhood depression. In the largest study of the use of antidepressants among children, Emslie and colleagues (86) compared fluoxetine with placebo and found that more than half of the fluoxetine group significantly benefited from treatment, whereas only 33 percent of the placebo group showed benefit.

In the only multisite controlled trial of SSRIs for childhood anxiety disorders, fluvoxamine was found to be superior to placebo in treating children with a diagnosis of social phobia, separation anxiety, or generalized anxiety disorder (87). In addition, several pharmacologic agents have been shown to be efficacious in the treatment of children or adolescents with a diagnosis of obsessive-compulsive disorder; these include SSRIs and tricyclic antidepressants (82,83). There is also evidence supporting the usefulness of antipsychotic medications for schizophrenia with onset in childhood or adolescence; however, data on long-term effectiveness and safety are lacking (16).

Unfortunately, despite the fact that in clinical practice it is common for medication treatments to be combined with psychosocial strategies, the literature on the impact of combined treatments for disorders other than ADHD is sparse. A large multi-site clinical trial of the efficacy of combined treatments for adolescent depression is under way and is expected to provide knowledge about treatment options in this area.

Potentially ineffective treatments. Recent efforts to identify empirically supported treatments for children have focused largely on the accumulation of supportive findings without an established procedure for dealing with null or even negative results (88). It is, in fact, just as important to identify treatments for which empirical studies consistently fail to show an effect on symptoms or even show worse outcomes for participants in the treatment group. *Youth Violence: A Report of the Surgeon General* (89) suggests that many of the services provided to delinquent juveniles have little or no evidence base.

Worse yet, a recent study indicated that peer-based, group-based interventions may actually increase behavioral problems among high-risk adolescents (90). For children who have disruptive-behavior disorders, there is no empirical justification for the use of nonbehavioral psychotherapies (91). For example, Pelham and colleagues (4), in their review of effective treatments for ADHD, found no empirical studies that tested the efficacy of many psychosocial treatments commonly used for ADHD, such as individual therapy and play therapy. In addition, although controlled treatment outcome studies have been conducted for cognitive therapy—for example, self-instruction, self-monitoring, and self-reinforcement—to treat children with a diagnosis of ADHD, these studies generally show no clinical or academic benefits from the treatment (92).

A third example of widely used but empirically unjustified services is institutional care—for example, hospitals, residential treatment centers, and group homes (13). Studies have shown that children who are placed in group homes do not maintain improvements once they return to the community (93). Yet group homes continue to be used in community practice.

A general conclusion from this review of evidence-based practices is that the literature on the efficacy of a range of child and adolescent treatments is uneven, although it is gaining strength for particular clinical syndromes. However, the evidence for the effectiveness of either clinical treatments or services within practice settings as opposed to research settings is still weak. Improving the evidence will require attention to service variables that tend to be neglected in most efficacy-based studies.

Presuppositions about evidence-based practice

Although the public health goal of developing a strong research base on effective services is to improve routine care, the implementation of research-based practice is not automatic. Rather, it requires adaptation of research design and methods to practice-related exigencies, as well as accommodation of practice settings to the incorporation of evidence-based practice. Other papers in this series have identified barriers to implementation of evidence-based practice. However, in the child and adolescent field, it is prudent to ask a different and prior set of questions. These questions have to do with whether empirically validated knowledge about treatments and services is ready to be implemented and, if not, why not. To think about these kinds of questions leads us to consider the models that typically guide development of evidence-based treatments and services and the extent to which implementation is justified given these models.

A presupposition of the evidence base is that its development has taken into account the fit between the treatment and the context of delivery. In fact, this fit has been attended to only rarely. One reason that efficacy studies, which constitute a significant portion of the evidence base in children's mental health, have not been readily deployed in service settings may be that the theory, methods, and models used to develop, refine, and test those treatments do not mesh well with the exigencies of clinic-based or community-based care (18).

The culture of psychological science as brought to bear on questions of the efficacy of treatments for children has typically involved conducting studies in controlled and somewhat rarefied environments, such as university laboratories. Over the past 40 years many controlled clinical trials and within-group studies have been published on the impact and efficacy of psychosocial treatments. Specific treatments have been identified for about two dozen clinical conditions in children. These studies have typically been conducted in or in close connection with university laboratories. Studies of conventional treatments delivered in clinics and clinical programs have demonstrated much weaker effects (94).

There has been an implicit assumption that once the laboratory studies of the efficacy of treatments have been completed, the results will be usable and relevant outside the laboratories. However, as has been noted repeatedly (13,18,94), the conditions under which most research is conducted differ in numerous ways from those under which everyday treatment is delivered. Such differences imply that treatments that have been developed through efficacy trials need to be adapted to clinics, schools, or other service settings. However, the differences also imply the opposite, namely, that the service settings or service practices themselves—that is, where, when, and how treatments are delivered—may have to adapt to accommodate delivery of evidence-based practices.

The model that has guided treatment development entails a series of controlled laboratory trials that focus on the efficacy of the treatment. Issues related to the effectiveness, dissemination, implementation, and deployment of treatments take place at the end of the testing process. This model tends to control experimentally the very "nuisance variables" that may need to be understood if treatments are to fit within clinic or community settings (18). These variables—such as comorbidity, parental substance abuse or pathology, life stresses that lead to early termination of treatment, reimbursement structures, service availability, and parental self-efficacy—may make or break the successful adoption of an evidence-based practice in a new practice setting.

Unfortunately, the development of the evidence base has rarely attended to such nuisance variables. Consequently, implementation of many treatments in clinic or community settings may be premature unless such factors are built into the long-term design and cumulative construction of new treatments and services. For example, studies of the development of combined treatments for children with depression who are first seen by primary care physicians should perhaps take into account service linkages with family practice physicians to treat maternal depression. Organizational variables, such as care management, that constrain or facilitate the ability of physicians to communicate with teachers about the impact of treatment on children should be taken into account at the front end of the treatment development cycle.

A second presupposition underlying evidence-based practice is that diffusion of the evidence base will be automatic once the strength of the evidence is ascertained. In fact, diffusion of innovative practice constitutes a researchable set of questions on its own. A major objective of most diffusion studies is to determine whether the practice is adopted as it was designed or adapted, whether the practice is sustained over time, and what factors influence sustainability (95). Diffusion is only beginning to be studied in the context of the mental health treatment of either children or adults. The literature on diffusion identifies individual and contextual factors that are potentially relevant to the effective diffusion of innovation in general, but not the specific factors most likely to predict adoption and implementation of a particular innovation, nor of a particular mental health treatment or service. Thus the evidence base needed to guide successful dissemination of effective treatments has yet to be developed (96).

The central problem is that treatments that have been validated in efficacy studies cannot be assumed to be effective when implemented under routine practice conditions. For example, the use of treatment manuals, special training for clinicians, and continual clinical monitoring to ensure treatment fidelity are characteristics of many research-based interventions but few community-based treatment practices. On the other hand, community treatment is characterized by heterogeneous populations and high caseloads, which are not features of most research-based studies (91). To enable a better fit between evidence-based treatments and community practice contexts will most likely require modifications of both the way in which evidence-based practice is created and modifi-

> *The central problem is that treatments that have been validated in efficacy studies cannot be assumed to be effective when implemented under routine practice conditions.*

cations in the service delivery settings. The variables at the interface that enable a better match have been described as issues of transportability (96). Features of research protocols and practice contexts that require modification—for example, the training and background of the practitioner, the setting, the organizational culture or context, and financing—and the kinds of modification required are variables that may well influence the portability of evidence-based practices and the adaptability of practice settings (18,41,96,97).

For example, transportability issues have been examined in studies of the promotion of physicians' use of new medications, devices, or procedures. Because most medical technologies must be approved by the FDA before being marketed, the efficacy of the technologies is not in question. However, questions about the fidelity of practitioners' implementation and how it may influence the effectiveness of the intervention cannot be assumed to have been studied. Although some studies of the impact of continuing education, academic detailing, training plus follow-up procedures, and hybrid strategies on physicians' implementation of new technologies have been conducted (98), their application to the dissemination of evidence-based practices in children's services is only now being studied (41), and these practices may well require adaptation.

Attention to the fit will require modification along a variety of dimensions, which differentiate research-based treatments from community practice. The dimensions include the intervention itself; the practitioners who deliver the intervention, including their clinical training, support, and monitoring; the client population (homogeneity or heterogeneity of syndromes); the characteristics of service delivery, such as the setting and the types of services available beyond the intervention; the organizational ethos—for example, the culture or climate in which practitioners provide services, which influences motivation, attitudes, and morale; and the service system, including referral and reimbursement mechanisms and interagency relations (96). The research base that constitutes evidence-based practice for child and adolescent mental health interventions has not typically assessed these dimensions of routine practice.

Finally, factors that predict successful dissemination of evidence-based practices may overlap with those that predict effective services, may be identical to them, or may be entirely different. For example, the organizational climate was found to be a strong predictor of psychosocial outcomes among children receiving casework services in a child welfare agency, and it appears to exert its influence through the motivational attitudes of casework therapists toward their work (99). Is organizational climate an important ingredient of uptake and dissemination? The answer to this question is not yet known. If climate is associated with interpersonal variables that predict the adoption of innovation, then manipulation of climate will be important to the eventual implementation of evidence-based practices. However, if the variables that predict uptake are more closely related to systemic or interpersonal dimensions rather than to organizational dimensions, then climate may not be the active agent for implementation.

Improving implementation of evidence-based practice

Improving implementation of evidence-based practice in children's services entails the adoption of new models of treatment development and augmentation of current effectiveness studies such that dimensions of typical practice are assessed and better understood. Weisz and Weersing (18) and Hoagwood and colleagues (41) have argued for the creation of clinic and community intervention development models that, in the initial piloting and manualization phase, attend to nuisance characteristics of the practice setting, such as practitioners' behaviors, organizational variables, and the characteristics of the community.

In addition, the new report of the National Institute of Mental Health's Advisory Council, titled *Blueprint for Change: Research on Child and Adolescent Mental Health* (100), describes a new cyclic model of treatment development that attends to service delivery issues at the outset. The report argues that attention to these contextual variables is necessary if the intervention is ultimately to be adopted. This model of intervention development is extremely challenging and not for the fainthearted. However, without such a revolution in treatment development, the best that can be hoped for is that evidence-based practices do not gather too much dust on academic shelves.

Conclusions

As the field of mental health services research expands, it will be important to take advantage of opportunities to study new services as they arise and to do so in a timely manner. On the basis of past performance, when treatments are developed and tested via the typical medical model, ten to 20 years may be required before the treatment can be understood in terms of its effects within a practice setting. As the Surgeon General's *National Action Agenda* for children's mental health (101) demonstrates, this time frame is impractical and inefficient if the goal of a public health science of children's services is to improve practice. Instead, a new model is needed that will encourage studies of the effectiveness of new treatments and services in the context of the practice setting in which the treatment or service is ultimately to be delivered. ◆

References

1. Kazdin AE: Current (lack of) status of theory in child and adolescent psychotherapy research. Journal of Clinical Child Psychology 28:533–543, 1999

2. Chambless DL, Sanderson WC, Shohman V, et al: An update on empirically validated therapies. Clinical Psychologist 49:5–18, 1996

3. Lonigan CJ, Elbert JC, Johnson SB: Empirically supported psychosocial interventions for children: an overview. Journal of Child Clinical Psychology 27:138–145, 1998

4. Pelham WE, Wheeler T, Chronis A: Empirically supported psychosocial treatments for attention deficit hyperactivity disorder. Journal of Child Clinical Psychology 27:190–205, 1998

5. Brestan EV, Eyberg SM: Effective psychosocial treatments of conduct-disordered children and adolescents: 29 years, 82 studies, and 5,272 kids. Journal of Child Clinical Psychology 27:180–189, 1998

6. Ollendick TH, King NJ: Empirically supported treatments for children with phobic and anxiety disorders. Journal of Child Clinical Psychology 27:156–167, 1998

7. Kaslow NJ, Thompson MP: Applying the criteria for empirically supported treatments to studies of psychosocial interventions for child and adolescent depression. Journal of Child Clinical Psychology 27:146–155, 1998

8. Weisz JR: Lab-clinic differences and what we can do about them: linking research and practice to enhance our public impact. Newsletter of the Division of Clinical Child Psychology, 2001, in press

9. Cochrane Collaboration and Health Information Research Unit: Preparing and Maintaining Systematic Reviews, in The Cochran Collaboration Handbook, edited by Oxman A. Oxford, England, Cochran Collaboration, 1994

10. Smith ML, Glass GV: Meta-analysis of psychotherapy outcomes studies. American Psychologist 32:752–760, 1977

11. Kazdin AE, Bass D, Ayers WA, et al: Empirical and clinical focus of child and adolescent psychotherapy research. Journal of Consulting Clinical Psychology 58:729–740, 1990

12. Weisz JR, Weiss B, Han SS, et al: Effects of psychotherapy with children and adolescents revisited: a meta-analysis of treatment outcome studies. Psychological Bulletin 117:450–468, 1995

13. Burns BJ, Hoagwood K, Mrazek P: Effective treatment for mental disorders in children and adolescents. Clinical Child and Family Psychology Review 2:199–254, 1999

14. Heneghan AM, Horwitz SM, Leventhal JM: Evaluating intensive family preservation programs: a methodologic review. Pediatrics 97:535–542, 1996

15. Rones M, Hoagwood K: School-based mental health services: a research review. Clinical Child and Family Psychology Review 3:223–241, 2000

16. Weisz JR, Jensen PS: Efficacy and effectiveness of child and adolescent psychotherapy and pharmacotherapy. Mental Health Services Research 1:125–158, 1999

17. Cook TF, Campbell DT: Quasi-Experimentation: Design and Analysis Issues for Field Settings. Chicago, Rand-McNally, 1979

18. Weisz JR, Weersing VR: Psychotherapy with children and adolescents: efficacy, effectiveness, and developmental concerns, in Rochester Symposium on Developmental Psychopathology, vol 9, Developmental Approaches to Prevention and Intervention. Edited by Cicchetti D, Toth SL. Rochester, NY, University of Rochester Press, 1999

19. Shadish W, Montgomery L, Wilson P, et al: The effects of family and marital psychotherapies: a meta-analysis. Journal of Consulting and Clinical Psychology 61:992–1002, 1993

20. Carr A: Evidence-based practice in family therapy and systemic consultation: I. child focused problems. Journal of Family Therapy 22:29–60, 2000

21. Cicchetti D, Tucker D: Development and self-regulatory structures of the mind. Development and Psychopathology 6:533–549, 1994

22. Yeh M, Weisz J: Why are we here at the clinic? Parent-child (dis)agreement on referral problems at outpatient treatment entry. Journal of Consulting and Clinical Psychology, in press

23. Jensen PS, Hoagwood K: The book of names: DSM-IV in context. Developmental Psychopathology 9:231–249, 1997

24. Burns BJ, Costello EJ, Angold A, et al:

Children's mental health service use across service sectors. Health Affairs 14(3):147–159, 1995

25. Kanner L: Child Psychiatry. Springfield, Ill, Thomas, 1935

26. Stroul BA, Friedman RM: Caring for severely emotionally disturbed children and youth: principles for a system of care. Children Today 17(4):15–17, 1988

27. Costello EJ, Angold A, Burns BJ, et al: The Great Smoky Mountains Study of Youth: goals, design, methods, and the prevalence of DSM-III-R disorders. Archives of General Psychiatry 53:1129–1136, 1996

28. Costello EJ, Angold A, Burns BJ, et al: The Great Smoky Mountains study of youth: functional impairment and serious emotional disturbance. Archives of General Psychiatry 53:1137–1143, 1996

29. Shaffer D, Fisher P, Dulcan MK, et al: The NIMH Diagnostic Interview Schedule for Children Version 2.3 (DISC-2.3): description, acceptability, prevalence rates, and performance in the MECA study. Journal of the American Academy of Child and Adolescent Psychiatry 35:865–877, 1996

30. Lahey BB, Flagg EW, Bird HR, et al: The NIMH methods for the epidemiology of child and adolescent mental disorders (MECA) study: background and methodology. Journal of the American Academy of Child and Adolescent Psychiatry 35:855–864, 1996

31. Leaf PJ, Alegria M, Cohen P, et al: Mental health service use in the community and schools: results from the four-community MECA study. Journal of the American Academy of Child and Adolescent Psychiatry 35:889–897, 1996

32. Bickman L: A continuum of care: more is not always better. American Psychologist 51:689–701, 1996

33. Bickman L: The Fort Bragg continuum of care for children and adolescents: mental health outcomes over 5 years. Journal of Consulting and Clinical Psychology 68:710–716, 2000

34. Weisz JR, Donenberg GR, Han SS, et al: Bridging the gap between laboratory and clinic in child and adolescent psychotherapy. Journal of Consulting and Clinical Psychology 63:688–701, 1995

35. Hoagwood K: Interpreting nullity: the Fort Bragg experiment—a comparative success or failure? American Psychologist 52:546–550, 1997

36. Henggeler SW, Rowland MD, Pickrel SG, et al: Investigating family-based alternatives to institution-based mental health services for youth: lessons learned from the pilot study of a randomized field trial. Journal of Clinical Child Psychology 26:226–233, 1997

37. Hoagwood K, Hibbs E, Brent D, et al: Introduction to the special section: efficacy and effectiveness in studies of child and adolescent psychotherapy. Journal of Consulting and Clinical Psychology 63:683–687, 1995

38. Hoagwood K, Jensen P, Petti T, et al: Outcomes of care for children and adolescents: a conceptual model. Journal of the American Academy of Child and Adolescent Psychiatry 35:1055–1063, 1996

39. Jensen PS, Hoagwood K, Petti T: Outcomes of mental health care for children and adolescents: II. literature review and application of a comprehensive model. Journal of the American Academy of Child and Adolescent Psychiatry 35:1064–1077, 1996

40. Burns BJ: A call for a mental health services research agenda for youth with serious emotional disturbance. Mental Health Services Research 1:5–20, 1999

41. Hoagwood K, Burns BJ, Weisz JR: A profitable conjunction: from research to practice in children's mental health, in Community-Based Interventions for Youth With Severe Emotional Disorders. Edited by Burns BJ, Hoagwood K. Oxford, New York, Oxford University Press, in press

42. National Advisory Mental Health Council's Clinical Treatment and Services Research Workgroup: Bridging Science to Service. Pub 99-4353. Rockville, Md, National Institute of Mental Health, 1999

43. Kazdin AE, Holland L, Crowley M: Family experiences of barriers to treatment and premature termination from child therapy. Journal of Consulting and Clinical Psychology 65:453–463, 1997

44. Armbruster P, Fallon T: Clinical, sociodemographic, and systems risk factors for attrition in a children's mental health clinic. American Journal of Orthopsychiatry 64:577–585, 1994

45. Kazdin AE: Premature termination from treatment among children referred for antisocial behavior. Journal of Clinical Child Psychology 31:415–425, 1993

46. Tuma JM: Mental health services for children. American Psychologist 44:188–189, 1989

47. Santisteban DA, Szapocznik J, Perez-Vidal A: Efficacy of intervention for engaging youth and families into treatment and some variables that may contribute to differential effectiveness. Journal of Family Psychology 10:35–44, 1996

48. Szapocznik J, Perez-Vidal A, Brickman AL, et al: Engaging adolescent drug abusers and their families in treatment: a strategic structural systems approach. Journal of Consulting and Clinical Psychology 56:552–557, 1988

49. McKay MM, McCadam K, Gonzales JJ: Addressing the barriers to mental health services for inner city children and their caretakers. Community Mental Health 32:353–361, 1996

50. Casey RJ, Berman JS: The outcome of psychotherapy with children. Psychological Bulletin 98: 388–400, 1985

51. Weisz JR, Weiss B, Alicke MD, et al: Effectiveness of psychotherapy with children and adolescents: a meta-analysis for clinicians. Journal of Consulting and Clinical Psychology 55:542–549, 1987

52. Weisz JR, Weiss B, Han SS, et al: Effects of psychotherapy with children and adolescents revisited: a meta-analysis of treatment outcome studies. Psychological Bulletin 117:450–468, 1995

53. Weisz JR, Donenberg GR, Han SS, et al: Bridging the gap between laboratory and clinic in child and adolescent psychotherapy. Journal of Consulting and Clinical Psychology 63:688–701, 1995

54. Burns BJ, Farmer EMZ, Angold A, et al: A randomised trial of case management for youths with serious emotional disturbance. Journal of Clinical Child Psychology 25:476–486, 1996

55. Evans ME, Huz S, McNulty T, et al: Child, family and system outcomes of intensive case management in New York State. Psychiatric Quarterly 67:273–287, 1996

56. Clarke HB, Prange M, Lee B, et al: An individualized wraparound process for children in foster care with emotional/behavioral disturbances: follow-up findings and implications from a controlled study, in Outcomes for Children and Youth With Behavioral and Emotional Disorders and Their Families. Edited by Epstein M, Kutash K, Duchnowski A. Austin, Tex, PRO-ED, 1998

57. Chamberlain P, Weinrott M: Specialized foster care: treating seriously emotionally disturbed children. Children Today 19(1):24–27, 1990

58. Clarke HB, Prange M, Lee B, et al: Improving adjustment outcomes for foster children with emotional and behavioral disorders: early findings from a controlled study on individualized services. Journal of Emotional and Behavioral Disorders 2:207–218, 1994

59. Chamberlain P, Reid JB: Using a specialized foster care community treatment model for children and adolescents leaving the state mental hospital. Journal of Community Psychology 19:266–276, 1991

60. Chamberlain P, Reid J: Comparison of two community alternatives to incarceration for chronic juvenile offenders. Journal of Consulting and Clinical Psychology 4:624–633, 1998

61. Schoenwald SK, Brown TL, Henggeler SW: Inside multisystemic therapy: therapist, supervisory, and program practices. Journal of Emotional and Behavioral Disorders 8:113–127, 2000

62. Henggeler SW, Melton GB, Smith LA, et al: Family preservation using multisystemic treatment: long-term follow-up to a clinical trial with serious juvenile offenders. Journal of Child and Family Studies 2:283–293, 1993

63. Borduin CM, Mann BJ, Cone LT, et al: Multisystemic treatment of serious juvenile offenders: long-term prevention of criminology and violence. Journal of Consulting and Clinical Psychology 63:569–578, 1995

64. Henggeler SW, Rowland MD, Randall J, et al: Home-based multisystemic therapy as an alternative to the hospitalization of youths in psychiatric crisis: clinical out-

comes. Journal of the American Academy of Child and Adolescent Psychiatry 38:1331–1339, 1999

65. Schoenwald SK, Ward DM, Henggeler SW, et al: MST vs hospitalization for crisis stabilization of youth: placement and service use 4 months post-referral. Mental Health Services Research 2:3–12, 2000

66. Borduin CM, Henggeler SW, Blaske DM, et al: Multisystemic treatment of adolescent sexual offenders. International Journal of Offender Therapy and Comparative Criminology 35:105–114, 1990

67. Brunk M, Henggeler SW, Whelan JP, et al: A comparison of multisystemic therapy and parent training in the brief treatment of child abuse and neglect. Journal of Consulting and Clinical Psychology 55:311–318, 1987

68. Dolan L, Kellam S, Brown C, et al: The short-term impact of two classroom-based preventive interventions on aggressive and shy behaviors and poor achievement. Journal of Applied Developmental Psychology 14:317–345, 1993

69. Kellam S, Rebok G, Ialongo N, et al: The course and malleability of aggressive behavior from early first grade into middle school: results of a developmental epidemiologically-based preventive trial. Journal of Child Psychology, Psychiatry, and the Allied Disciplines 35:259–281, 1994

70. Fuchs D, Fuchs L, Bahr M: Mainstream assistance teams: a scientific basis for the art of consultation. Exceptional Children 57:128–139, 1990

71. Clarke G, Hawkins W, Murphy M, et al: Targeted prevention of unipolar depressive disorder in an at-risk sample of high school adolescents: a randomized trial of a group cognitive intervention. Journal of the American Academy of Child and Adolescent Psychiatry 34:312–321, 1995

72. Gillham J, Reivich K, Jaycox L, et al: Prevention of depressive symptoms in school children: two-year follow-up. Psychological Science 6:343–351, 1995

73. Reid J, Eddy M, Fetrow R, et al: Description and immediate impacts of a preventive intervention for conduct problems. American Journal of Community Psychology 27:483–517, 1999

74. Jensen PS, Bhatara V, Vietello B, et al: Psychoactive medication prescribing practices for US children: gaps between research and clinical practice. Journal of the American Academy of Child and Adolescent Psychiatry 38:557–565, 1999

75. Zito JM, Safer DJ, dosReis S, et al: Trends in the prescribing of psychotropic medications to preschoolers. JAMA 283:1025–1060, 2000

76. Hughes CW, Emslie GJ, Crismon ML, et al: The Texas Children's Medication Algorithm Project: report of the Texas Consensus Conference Panel on Medication Treatment of Childhood Major Depressive Disorder. Journal of the American Academy of Child and Adolescent Psychiatry 38:1442–1454, 1999

77. MTA Cooperative Group: A 14-month randomized clinical trial of treatment strategies for attention-deficit/hyperactivity disorder. Archives of General Psychiatry 56:1073–1086, 1999

78. Jobson KO, Potter WZ: International Psychopharmacology Algorithm Project report. Psychopharmacology Bulletin 31:457–459, 1995

79. Special section on current knowledge and unmet needs in pediatric psychopharmacology. Journal of the American Academy of Child and Adolescent Psychiatry 38:501–565, 1999

80. Greenhill LL, Halperin JM, Abikoff H: Stimulant medications. Journal of the American Academy of Child and Adolescent Psychiatry 38:503–512, 1999

81. Ryan ND, Bhatara VS, Perel JM: Mood stabilizers in children and adolescents. Journal of the American Academy of Child and Adolescent Psychiatry 38:529–536, 1999

82. Emslie GJ, Walkup JT, Pliszka SR, et al: Nontricyclic antidepressants: current trends in children and adolescents. Journal of the American Academy of Child and Adolescent Psychiatry 38:517–528, 1999

83. Geller B, Reising D, Leonard HL, et al: Critical review of tricyclic antidepressant use in children and adolescents. Journal of the American Academy of Child and Adolescent Psychiatry 38:513–516, 1999

84. Campbell M, Rapoport JL, Simpson GM: Antipsychotics in children and adolescents. Journal of the American Academy of Child and Adolescent Psychiatry 38:537–545, 1999

85. Riddle MA, Bernstein GA, Cook EH, et al: Anxiolytics, adrenergic agents, and naltrexone. Journal of the American Academy of Child and Adolescent Psychiatry 38:546–556, 1999

86. Emslie GJ, Rush AJ, Weinberg WA, et al: A double-blind, randomized, placebo-controlled trial of fluoxetine in children and adolescents with depression. Archives of General Psychiatry 54:1031–1037, 1997

87. Vitiello B, Bhatara VS, Jensen PS: Current knowledge and unmet needs in pediatric psychopharmacology. Journal of Abnormal Child Psychology 22:560–568, 1999

88. Weisz JR, Hawley KM: Finding, evaluating, refining, and applying empirically supported treatments for children and adolescents.

Journal of Clinical Child Psychology 27:206–216, 1998

89. Youth Violence: A Report of the Surgeon General. Washington, DC, US Public Health Service, 2001

90. Dishion TJ, McCord J, Poulin F: When interventions harm: peer groups and problem behavior. American Psychologist 54:755–765, 1999

91. Weisz JR, Donenberg GR, Han SS, et al: Bridging the gap between laboratory and clinic in child and adolescent psychotherapy. Journal of Consulting and Clinical Psychology 63:688–701, 1995

92. Abikoff H, Gittelman R: Hyperactive children treated with stimulants: is cognitive training a useful adjunct? Archives of General Psychiatry 42:953–961, 1985

93. Kirigin KA, Braukmann CJ, Atwater JD, et al: An evaluation of teaching-family (achievement place) group homes for juvenile offenders. Journal of Applied Behavior Analysis 15:1–16, 1982

94. Weisz JR, Weiss B, Donenberg GR: The lab versus the clinic: effects of child and adolescent psychotherapy. American Psychologist 47:1578–1585, 1992

95. Van de Ven AH, Polley DE, Garud R, et al: The Innovation Journey. Oxford, NY: Oxford University Press, 1999

96. Schoenwald SK, Hoagwood K: Effectiveness, transportability, and dissemination of interventions: what matters when? Psychiatric Services 52:1190–1197, 2001

97. Norquist G, Lebowitz B, Hyman S: Expanding the frontier of treatment research. Available at http://journals.apa.org/prevention/volume2/pre0020001a.html, 2000

98. Wensing M, van der Weijden T, Grol R: Implementing guidelines and innovations in general practice: which interventions are effective? British Journal of General Practice 48:991–997, 1998

99. Glisson C, Hemmelgarn A: The effects of organizational climate and interorganizational coordination on the quality of outcomes of children's service systems. Child Abuse and Neglect 22:401–421, 1998

100. National Institute of Mental Health Advisory Council Workgroup Report: Blueprint for Change: Research on Child and Adolescent Mental Health. Bethesda, Maryland, National Institute of Mental Health, 2001

101. Report of the Surgeon General's Conference on Children's Mental Health: A National Action Agenda. Washington, DC, US Public Health Service, 2000

Evidence-Based Practices in Geriatric Mental Health Care

Stephen J. Bartels, M.D.
Aricca R. Dums, B.A.
Thomas E. Oxman, M.D.
Lon S. Schneider, M.D.
Patricia A. Areán, Ph.D.
George S. Alexopoulos, M.D.
Dilip V. Jeste, M.D.

The past decade has seen dramatic growth in research on treatments for the psychiatric problems of older adults. An emerging evidence base supports the efficacy of geriatric mental health interventions. The authors provide an overview of the evidence base for clinical practice. They identified three sources of evidence—evidence-based reviews, meta-analyses, and expert consensus statements—on established and emerging interventions for the most common disorders of late life, which include depression, dementia, substance abuse, schizophrenia, and anxiety. The most extensive research support was found for the effectiveness of pharmacological and psychosocial interventions for geriatric major depression and for dementia. Less is known about the effectiveness of treatments for the other disorders, although emerging evidence is promising for selected interventions. Empirical support was also found for the effectiveness of community-based, multidisciplinary, geriatric psychiatry treatment teams. The authors discuss barriers to implementing evidence-based practices in the mental health service delivery system for older adults. They describe approaches to overcoming these barriers that are based on the findings of research on practice change and dissemination. Successful approaches to implementing change in the practices of providers emphasize moving beyond traditional models of continuing medical education to include educational techniques that actively involve the learner, as well as systems change interventions such as integrated care management, implementation toolkits, automated reminders, and decision support technologies. The anticipated growth in the population of older persons with mental disorders underscores the need for a strategy to facilitate the systematic and effective implementation of evidence-based practices in geriatric mental health care.

Dr. Bartels and Dr. Oxman are affiliated with the department of psychiatry at Dartmouth Medical School in Hanover, New Hampshire. They and Ms. Dums are affiliated with the New Hampshire–Dartmouth Psychiatric Research Center in Lebanon, New Hampshire. Dr. Schneider is with the department of psychiatry and behavioral sciences at the Keck School of Medicine at the University of Southern California, Los Angeles. Dr. Areán is with the department of psychiatry at the University of California, San Francisco. Dr. Alexopoulos is with the department of psychiatry at the Weill Medical College of Cornell University in White Plains, New York. Dr. Jeste is affiliated with the department of psychiatry at the University of California, San Diego, and the San Diego Veterans Affairs Medical Center. Send correspondence to Dr. Bartels at the New Hampshire–Dartmouth Psychiatric Research Center, 2 Whipple Place, Suite 202, Lebanon, New Hampshire 03766 (e-mail, stephen.j.bartels@dartmouth.edu). This article was originally published in the November 2002 issue of Psychiatric Services.

Treatment of mental disorders among older Americans has become a major public health need. The number of people over the age of 65 with psychiatric disorders will more than double by the year 2030, from 7 million in 2000 to 15 million (1). The past decade has seen dramatic growth in research on the causes and treatments of the psychiatric problems of older adults.

In this article we provide an overview of empirically validated treatments as reflected in systematic reviews of the literature on geriatric mental health interventions. Three types of evaluations of the literature on major geriatric mental health disorders are summarized: systematic evidence-based-practice reviews, meta-analytic studies, and expert consensus statements. Next we summarize major barriers to the dissemination and implementation of these practices. Finally, we describe possible strategies for disseminating and implementing evidence-based practices in geriatric mental health care.

An impending public health crisis

At least one in five people over the age of 65 suffers from a mental disorder (1). By 2030 the number of persons with psychiatric disorders in this older group will equal or exceed the number with such disorders in younger age groups (age 18 to 29 or age 30 to 44) (1). Despite the growing requirement for mental health services for older persons, there is substantial unmet need. The 1999 Surgeon General's report on mental health (2), the Administration on Aging's 2001 report (3), and an expert consensus statement (1) underscore the need to plan for the provision of services for the growing number of elderly persons with major mental disorders.

Older adults with mental disorders are more likely than younger adults to receive inappropriate or inadequate treatments (4). Bridging the gap between research and clinical services has been identified as one of the most important priorities in health care (5,6). Among the greatest challenges is the "expertise gap" that affects clinicians practicing in routine settings. This gap is the result of inadequate training in geriatric care and a failure to incorporate contemporary research findings and evidence-based practices into usual care.

Evidence-based practices

Many of the underlying principles of evidence-based practice reflect Cochrane's (7) assertion three decades ago that our limited health care resources should be applied to providing interventions that have proven effectiveness based on well-designed evaluation trials, with emphasis on randomized controlled trials. In this respect, evidence-based practice draws heavily on the use of external evidence to support clinical judgment (8). Criteria for evidence-based practices define different levels of empirical support based on the quality of the data (8,9). The specific criteria vary, but the underlying principles for identifying effective treatments are the same: support must be derived from well-designed controlled trials, and findings must be replicated by different investigators with sufficiently large samples from which results can be generalized (8,9).

In the hierarchy of evidence-based reviews of the literature, the highest level is occupied by systematic reviews that evaluate the level of evidence with strict criteria and by aggregate meta-analyses of all relevant randomized controlled trials (8). The following section provides an overview of the evidence base for geriatric mental health interventions derived from this standard of empirical evidence. This overview of published evidence-based reviews and

meta-analyses is not intended to be an exhaustive summary of the research literature but rather a starting point that defines geriatric mental health treatments with proven effectiveness.

English-language review articles that examined the effectiveness of geriatric mental health services were identified for the most common psychiatric problems among older adults: depression, dementia, alcohol abuse, schizophrenia, and anxiety disorders (10) through searches of MEDLINE, PsycINFO, and the Cochrane Library. Disorders for which we were unable to identify evidence-based reviews, meta-analyses, or consensus statements specifically targeting older adults, such as bipolar disorder, were not considered.

Searches were conducted of articles published through the year 2001, including but not limited to the terms evidence-based review, meta-analysis, consensus statement, consensus review, and review article. The evidence-based reviews included were those that systematically categorized studies and applied strict criteria for rating the level of evidence. The meta-analyses included were those that described and applied standardized meta-analytic statistical procedures. Expert consensus statements were included that described a systematic method of obtaining, evaluating, and summarizing expert consensus opinion on effective treatments.

This approach identified eight evidence-based reviews, 26 meta-analytic studies, and 12 expert consensus statements, which are summarized in the five tables. The first two categories were used to determine the evidence base defining effective treatments and services, and the third was included to provide a synopsis of effective treatments and best practices from the perspective of researchers and clinicians.

Geriatric depression

As shown in Table 1, there is general agreement on the effectiveness of antidepressants for geriatric depression (11–22). In general, more than half of older adults treated with antidepressants experience at least a 50 percent reduction in depressive symptoms (12). However, a recent meta-analysis of antidepressant studies that includ-

ed all age groups found that antidepressants offer only a 20 percent (2 points) greater reduction in scores on the Hamilton Rating Scale for Depression compared with placebo. This analysis suggests that placebo medication combined with visits by the prescribing physician may account for 80 percent of the effect of antidepressants (23). In addition, the comparative efficacy and tolerability of different classes of antidepressants remain controversial. Meta-analyses have not shown significant differences between the selective serotonin reuptake inhibitors (SSRIs) and the older tricyclic agents in terms of efficacy or treatment dropout from adverse effects. In contrast, expert consensus statements recommend SSRIs as first-line agents for geriatric depression and suggest avoiding tertiary amine antidepressants, such as amitriptyline, imipramine, and doxepin, because of the serious side effects, including cardiovascular and anticholinergic side effects, associated with their use (18–22).

Although the meta-analyses did not find a difference in tolerability between SSRIs and tricyclics on the basis of rates of discontinuation due to side effects, clinically significant differences may still be present. For example, common reasons for discontinuing SSRIs include sleep disturbance, gastrointestinal distress, anxiety, headaches, and weight loss, whereas common complications of tricyclic agents include more worrisome side effects, such as postural hypotension and arrhythmia (14).

Table 2 summarizes the efficacy of psychosocial treatments for geriatric depression (11,14,16,18,20–22,24–30). In general, cognitive therapy, behavioral therapy, and cognitive-behavioral therapy have the greatest empirical support for effectiveness in the treatment of geriatric depression. A variety of other psychosocial interventions are likely to be efficacious among older adults, including problem-solving therapy, interpersonal therapy, brief psychodynamic therapy, and reminiscence therapy. Moreover, it is likely that a combination of pharmacological and psychosocial interventions is more effective than either intervention alone in preventing

Table 1

Pharmacological treatments for geriatric depression

Evidence source and reference	Comments
Evidence-based reviews	
Thorpe et al., 2001 (11)	18 studies rated using standard guideline development criteria to determine preferred treatments. First-line treatments include bupropion, citalopram, fluvoxamine, mirtazapine, moclobemide, nefaxodone, paroxetine, sertraline, and venlafaxine. Electroconvulsive therapy (ECT) is effective.
Meta-analyses	
Wilson et al., 2001 (12)	17 randomized controlled trials (RCTs) reviewed of community patients and inpatients over age 55. Tricyclics are effective. Selective serotonin reuptake inhibitors (SSRIs) and monoamine oxidase inhibitors (MAOIs) are likely to be effective. Discontinuation rates are similar across agents and placebo.
Anderson, 2000 (13)	11 RCTs support efficacy and tolerability for SSRIs and tricyclics among depressed adults over age 65. No significant difference in efficacy or tolerability between SSRIs and tricyclics.
Gerson et al., 1999 (14)	41 RCTs reviewed for treatment of major or unipolar depression for patients over age 55. Tricyclics, SSRIs, and "other" antidepressants are superior to placebo. Comparable efficacy and tolerability between tricyclics and SSRIs, but patients taking "other" antidepressants had lower dropout rates due to side effects.
Mulrow et al., 1999 (15)	27 RCTs reviewed for treatment of major depression among outpatients over age 60. SSRIs, newer SSRIs, and tricyclics are superior to placebo. Efficacy and discontinuation rates do not differ between classes.
McCusker et al., 1998 (16)	26 controlled studies reviewed for treatment of depression among adults aged 55 and over in community, outpatient, or nursing home settings. Heterocyclics and SSRIs are equally effective.
Mittmann et al., 1997 (17)	49 RCTs evaluated through 1996 for treatment of moderate or severe major or unipolar depression among patients over age 60. SSRIs, newer SSRIs, tricyclics, and MAOIs have similar efficacy, safety, and tolerability.
Expert consensus statements	
Alexopoulos et al., 2001 (18)	SSRIs preferred for all depression types; especially favorable results for citalopram, sertraline, and paroxetine. SSRIs or venlafaxine plus psychotherapy preferred for major depression. SSRIs plus psychotherapy preferred for mild depression or dysthymia. SSRIs or venlafaxine plus an atypical antipsychotic preferred for psychotic major depression. ECT is effective and a first-line treatment.
Mulsant et al., 2001 (19)	SSRIs recommended as first-line antidepressants. Patients unable to tolerate or unresponsive to antidepressants can be switched to another agent or be treated with interpersonal psychotherapy.
American Society of Health-System Pharmacists, 1998 (20)	Similar efficacy for different classes of antidepressants. Selection based on side effect profile, prior treatment response, type of depression, severity of symptoms, and concurrent drug therapy.
Lebowitz et al., 1997 (21)	SSRIs and tricyclics have comparable efficacy. However, SSRIs may be preferred because they are easier to use, require less dosage adjustment, and have more favorable side effect profiles.
National Institutes of Health, 1992 (22)	Most antidepressants are equally effective. Amitriptyline and imipramine should be avoided. Newer antidepressants favored due to decreased anticholinergic and cardiovascular side effects. Treatment should be continued at a sufficient dose for six to 12 weeks.

recurrence of major depression, although replication of these findings is warranted (2,18). Expert consensus findings recommend the combined use of antidepressants and psychotherapy in the treatment of late-life depression, especially for episodes in which there is a clearly identified psychosocial stressor (18). Finally, a meta-analysis that compared the rates of response to pharmacological and psychological treatments of depression among patients over the age of 55 found similar effectiveness for antidepressants (tricyclics and SSRIs) and psychotherapeutic interventions (cognitive-behavioral, behavioral, and psychodynamic therapies), although firm conclusions are not possible given the small number of studies (14).

Evidence-based reviews of interventions for geriatric depression primarily address major depression, with

Table 2

Psychosocial treatments for geriatric depression

Evidence source and reference	Comments
Evidence-based reviews Laidlaw, 2001 (24)	6 meta-analyses and 10 outcome studies evaluated cognitive therapy for older adults with depression. It is effective for geriatric depression.
Thorpe et al., 2001 (11)	4 studies evaluated using standardized procedures to evaluate efficacy. Cognitive-behavioral therapy and interpersonal therapy for mild to moderate depression have the most support among psychotherapies.
Gatz et al., 1998 (25)	21 studies evaluated using evidence-based criteria to determine efficacy. Cognitive therapy, behavior therapy, cognitive-behavioral therapy, brief psychodynamic therapy, life review, reminiscence therapy are "likely to be effective."

Meta-analyses
  Pinquart and Soerensen,
    2001 (26)
	122 controlled psychotherapeutic studies compared; each had an untreated control group with depression (mean age of over 55). Cognitive-behavioral therapy, brief psychodynamic therapy, and supported psychotherapy are effective.

Gerson et al., 1999 (14)	4 randomized controlled trials (RCTs) evaluated, comparing treatment response and tolerability for people over age 55. Cognitive-behavioral therapy, brief psychodynamic therapy, and drug treatment have similar efficacy and tolerability.
Cuijpers, 1998 (27)	14 studies evaluated of the effectiveness of outpatient psychotherapy for adults over age 55, including 12 RCTs. Comparable efficacy found for cognitive-behavioral therapy, problem-solving therapy, behavior therapy, supportive therapy, reminiscence therapy, and brief psychodynamic therapy.
McCusker et al., 1998 (16)	14 controlled studies evaluated for treatment of depression in adults age over age 55 in community, outpatient, and nursing home settings. Cognitive therapy and behavior therapy better than no treatment but not better than a similar amount of nontherapeutic contact or attention given to a control group.
Engels and Verney, 1997 (28)	17 studies assessed for treatment of depression; age range, 52 to 81 years; mean age, 69 years. Treatment is more effective than placebo or no treatment. Behavior therapy and cognitive therapy are equally effective, and more effective than cognitive-behavioral therapy and brief psychodynamic psychotherapy. Individual therapy is more effective than group therapy.
Koder et al., 1996 (29)	7 studies evaluated of cognitive therapy for older people; mean age range, 65 to 70 years. It is more effective than wait-list control group and may be more effective than behavior therapy or brief psychodynamic psychotherapy.
Scogin and McElreath, 1994 (30)	17 studies of the efficacy of psychosocial treatments for depressed patients; mean age, 62 to 85 years. Comparable efficacy of cognitive therapy, behavior therapy, interpersonal therapy, and supportive therapy.
Expert consensus statements Alexopoulos et al., 2001 (18)	Preferred psychotherapies include cognitive-behavioral therapy, supportive psychotherapy, problem-solving therapy, and interpersonal therapy. Psychoeducation and family counseling are also supported.
American Society of Health- System Pharmacists, 1998 (20)	Cognitive therapy, behavior therapy, and interpersonal therapy are effective as primary interventions for older adults with mild to moderate depression or can be used in combination with pharmacotherapy.
Lebowitz et al., 1997 (21)	Cognitive-behavioral therapy, behavior therapy, problem-solving therapy, and interpersonal therapy are effective alone and in combination with drug treatments.
National Institutes of Health, 1992 (22)	Psychosocial treatments are indicated in patients who do not tolerate or accept biological treatments. Cognitive-behavioral therapy, behavior therapy, interpersonal therapy, and brief psychodynamic psychotherapy are moderately effective.

little attention to the treatment of associated conditions such as minor depression or suicidal behaviors. The number of studies addressing the treatment of minor depression among older persons is limited. For example, the results of randomized placebo-controlled studies of SSRIs in the treatment of older adults with minor depression suggest only modest benefits (31). In addition, little is known about the efficacy of interventions in

Table 3

Pharmacological and psychosocial treatment for cognitive symptoms of dementia

Evidence source and reference	Comments
Evidence-based reviews	
Brodaty et al., 2001 (33)	7 meta-analyses or systematic reviews and 21 studies evaluated using U.S. Food and Drug Administration standards. Cholinesterase inhibitors supported for people with mild to moderate dementia. Ginkgo biloba has a small effect on cognitive performance, but evidence is weaker than for cholinesterase inhibitors.
Doody et al., 2001 (34)	82 studies evaluated using standardized criteria to assign levels of evidence. Cholinesterase inhibitors have modest benefit for patients with Alzheimer's disease; vitamin E likely delays clinical worsening; selegiline, other antioxidants, and anti-inflammatories require further study. Estrogen should not be prescribed to treat Alzheimer's disease.
Kasl-Godley and Gatz, 2000 (35)	22 studies evaluated to determine empirical support for reality orientation therapy and memory training. Memory training may optimize remaining ability. Reality orientation is useful for interpersonal but not cognitive functioning.
Gatz et al., 1998 (25)	18 studies evaluated using evidence-based criteria. Memory and cognitive retraining programs may be effective in slowing decay of skills. Reminiscence is not effective. Reality orientation may improve orientation but does not generalize to other settings.
American Psychiatric Association, 1997 (36)	8 randomized controlled trials (RCTs), 5 for tacrine and 3 for donepezil, support modest improvement of cognition with cholinesterase inhibitors. Possible delay of poor outcomes suggested by 1 RCT of vitamin E and 7 RCTS of selegiline. No indication for ergot mesylate in treatment of Alzheimer's disease based on 7 RCTs.
National Institute for Clinical Excellence, 2001 (37)	5 RCTs for donepezil, 5 for rivastigmine, and 3 for galantamine and 3 systematic reviews for donepezil, 3 for rivastigmine, and 1 for galantamine. All agents significantly improved cognitive functioning.
Meta-analyses	
Birks and Flicker, 2001 (38)	15 RCTs evaluated for selegiline (a selective monoamine oxidase inhibitor at low doses) administered to patients with dementia for more than 1 day. Improvement in several memory tests, yet not enough evidence to recommend use in routine practice.
Birks et al., 2001 (39)	8 RCTs of donepezil (a cholinesterase inhibitor) evaluated for patients with mild to moderate Alzheimer's disease treated for 12, 24, and 52 weeks. Modest improvements in cognitive functioning and global clinical ratings compared with placebo.
Fioravanti and Flicker, 2001 (40)	11 RCTs of nicergoline (an ergot derivative) assessed. Potential benefit found for cognitive and behavioral symptoms in vascular dementia, but is associated with an increased risk of adverse effects. No definitive studies of use in Alzheimer's disease.
Fioravanti and Yanagi, 2001 (41)	12 RCTs of cytidinediphosphocholine (a phosphatidylcholine precursor) assessed. Some evidence suggests positive short-term effects on memory, behavior, and global impression.
Olin and Schneider, 2001 (42)	7 RCTs evaluated of galantamine (a cholinesterase inhibitor) for mild to moderate Alzheimer's disease administered for 3 to 6 months. Galantamine improves global ratings, cognition, activities of daily living, and behavior with effect and tolerability comparable to that of other cholinesterase inhibitors.
Spector et al., 2001 (43)	6 RCTs of reality orientation assessed. Some evidence that reality orientation benefits cognitive and behavioral symptoms of dementia.
Birks et al., 2000 (44)	7 RCTs of rivastigmine (a cholinesterase inhibitor) evaluated for patients with Alzheimer's disease treated for more than 2 weeks. Rivastigmine is more effective than placebo in improving cognitive function and activities of daily living.
Higgins and Flicker, 2000 (45)	12 RCTs of lecithin (a dietary source of choline) evaluated. Evidence does not support the use of lecithin in the treatment of dementia or cognitive impairment.
Qizilbash et al., 1998 (46)	12 RCTs of tacrine (a cholinesterase inhibitor) assessed. It reduces deterioration in cognitive performance over the first 3 months of treatment and may result in global improvement.
Oken et al., 1998 (47)	4 RCTs of gingko biloba for patients with Alzheimer's disease. Small effect on cognitive function over 4 to 6 months of treatment. No significant adverse effects.
Expert consensus statements	
Patterson et al., 1999 (48)	12 studies reviewed supporting an evidence-based consensus statement. Donepezil improves cognitive functioning in mild to moderate dementia. Insufficient evidence to recommend vitamin E or ginkgo biloba for treatment or prevention of Alzheimer's disease.
Small et al., 1997 (49)	Cholinesterase inhibitors slow cognitive decline. Evidence for other agents is inconclusive. Reality orientation and memory retraining may be beneficial, but the associated risks of frustration and depression may outweigh the small benefits.

Table 4

Pharmacological and psychosocial treatment for behavioral symptoms of dementia

Evidence source and reference	Comments
Evidence-based reviews Doody et al., 2001 (34)	94 studies of pharmacological and psychosocial treatment evaluated. Antipsychotics are effective for agitation or psychosis when environmental approaches fail; antidepressants are effective in depression with dementia. Behavior modification and skills training can also be effective.
Kasl-Godley and Gatz, 2000 (35)	22 studies of psychosocial and behavioral interventions evaluated. Reminiscence and life review result in small improvements in interpersonal behavior. Support groups and cognitive therapy or behavior therapy help build coping skills and reduce distress. Behavioral approaches are helpful with early-stage dementia.
Gatz et al., 1998 (25)	12 studies of psychosocial and behavioral interventions evaluated using *DSM* criteria. Reinforcement, extinction, and stimulus control are effective, although they have a limited scope. Environmental approaches, such as milieu therapy, a token economy, and environmental modifications, are effective.
American Psychiatric Association, 1997 (36)	7 randomized controlled trials (RCTs) of pharmacological interventions reviewed. Modest improvement of agitation and psychosis in dementia with conventional antipsychotics. 7 RCTs of benzodiazepines show improvement of agitation compared with placebo but not better than antipsychotics. Insufficient data to assess atypical antipsychotics or anticonvulsants. 5 RCTs of antidepressant treatment of depression in dementia suggest benefit, although limited by small samples and by selection criteria.
Meta-analyses Kirchner et al., 2001 (59)	12 RCTs evaluated for thioridazine (a conventional neuroleptic). No evidence to support its use in the treatment of dementia. Only positive effect was reduction in anxiety.
Lonergan et al., 2001 (60)	5 RCTs of haloperidol (a conventional neuroleptic) assessed for agitation in dementia. Evidence supports its use in the control of aggression. No evidence for improvement in other forms of agitation, and there are frequent side effects.
Olin et al., 2001 (61)	19 RCTs evaluated for hydergine (an ergoloid mesylate). Significant treatment effects when assessed by either global ratings or comprehensive rating scales. Because of uncertainty in diagnostic criteria, the efficacy of hydergine for dementia is not clear.
Lanctot et al., 1998 (62)	16 RCTs (1966 to 1997) of conventional neuroleptics. No difference in efficacy between different agents. Conventional neuroleptics have modest efficacy compared with placebo.
Schneider et al., 1990 (63)	7 RCTs of conventional neuroleptics (1960 to 1982). They are modestly more effective than placebo, but the effect size was small (r=.18). No single agent is better than another.
Expert consensus statements Herrmann, 2001 (64)	Nonpharmacological approaches favored as first-line treatment for behavioral symptoms of dementia, although high-quality research is limited. Atypical antipsychotics, antidepressants, and anticonvulsants are modestly effective in reducing behavioral symptoms. Benzodiazepines may be used if necessary. Pharmacotherapy should be monitored for effectiveness and side effects.
Patterson et al., 1999 (48)	24 studies reviewed supporting an evidence-based consensus statement. Environmental and behavioral modifications should be first-line treatments for behavioral problems. If medications are required, low doses of antipsychotics, a selective serotonin reuptake inhibitor (SSRI), or trazodone should be considered.
Alexopoulos et al., 1998 (65)	Combined medication and environmental interventions favored as first-line treatment for agitation in dementia. Mild agitation treatment: structured routines, reassurance, and socialization; severe agitation treatment: supervision and environmental safety. Both should include education and support for family and caregivers. Preferred medication varies with presenting conditions: For psychosis, risperidone or a conventional, high-potency antipsychotic; for depression, an antidepressant alone (sertraline or paroxetine); for aggression and anger, divalproex, risperidone, a conventional, high potency antipsychotic, an SSRI, trazodone, or buspirone.
Small et al., 1997 (49)	SSRIs favored as first-line treatments for depression in dementia. Tricyclics are effective but have greater side effects. Antipsychotics are modestly effective for behavioral problems and psychotic symptoms. More studies are needed to establish efficacy of other agents. Psychotherapy may decrease behavioral problems and improve mood.

Table 5

Pharmacological and psychosocial treatment for geriatric alcohol abuse

Evidence source and reference

Evidence-based reviews Gatz et al., 1998 (25)	3 studies evaluated using evidence-based criteria to determine treatment efficacy. Reminiscence, age segregation, and a supportive climate are promising but require further study.
Expert consensus statements Center for Substance Abuse Treatment, 1998 (72)	Brief interventions, motivational counseling, and family interventions recommended. Treatment principles: age specific; supportive group treatment; focus on coping with depression, loneliness, and loss; rebuilding social support network; pace and content appropriate for older persons; clinicians interested and experienced in older adult populations; linkage with medical and aging services, case management, and referral sources.
Council on Scientific Affairs, 1996 (73)	Detoxification should occur in a hospital setting and medications should be carefully monitored. Age-specific groups and programs that emphasize social relationships and positive aspects of a patient's life have better outcomes for older adults.

preventing suicidal behaviors among older adults, even though the rate of suicide among older adults is greater than in any other age group (32). An evidence-based review of the literature suggests that the only supported preventive intervention for late-life suicide is the identification and effective treatment of depression (32).

In summary, there is a well-substantiated evidence base supporting the efficacy of antidepressants and cognitive, behavioral, and cognitive-behavioral therapy in the acute and short-term treatment of geriatric major depression. However, caution is indicated in interpreting the results of individual studies that report the superiority of one treatment over another—for example, SSRIs over tricyclic agents—because of the potential sources of bias, which include industry sponsorship of clinical trials, sample selection, and study design.

Dementia

Evidence of treatment effectiveness for dementia can be separated into studies of cognitive symptoms, such as problems with memory, language, and abstraction, and studies of behavioral symptoms, such as agitation, psychosis, and depression.

Cognitive symptoms

As shown in Table 3 (25,33–49), for patients with mild to moderate dementia associated with Alzheimer's disease, evidence-based reviews and meta-analyses agree on the effective-

ness of cholinesterase inhibitors compared with placebo in modestly reducing the rate of decline or enhancing cognitive functioning over the course of six to 12 months. In addition, evidence is emerging that cholinesterase inhibitors may be effective in delaying nursing home placement (50) and that they may improve cognitive functioning in severe Alzheimer's dementia (51) and in some non-Alzheimer's dementias (52). Selegiline may also be used, although it has a less favorable risk-benefit ratio and less supporting evidence (34,38). In the one placebo-controlled trial of vitamin E, no significant differences were found in cognitive signs and symptoms, although vitamin E minimally slowed progression to institutionalization (53). The effectiveness of other antioxidants, anti-inflammatories, estrogen replacement, ginkgo biloba extracts, and other agents is not supported by evidence. However, research on the pharmacotherapy of Alzheimer's disease is a rapidly advancing field, and a variety of multicenter trials that hold promise for expanding the array of available evidence-based treatments are under way.

In general, psychosocial treatments for the cognitive symptoms of dementia are not effective (25,34,35,49). A review of the empirical evidence for cognitive retraining programs and reality orientation suggests that these interventions may temporarily improve cognitive, behavioral, and functional skills, but compelling evidence of sustained benefit is lacking (25,43).

In summary, despite a traditionally pessimistic view of treatments for dementia, there is an emerging evidence base supporting modest effectiveness of cholinesterase inhibitors in temporarily decreasing cognitive decline and enhancing cognitive functioning for mild to moderate Alzheimer's dementia over six to 12 months.

Behavioral symptoms

Thirty to 40 percent of persons with Alzheimer's dementia experience behavioral symptoms, including agitation, psychosis, and depression, at some point during the disease (49). Limited research consisting of individual randomized placebo-controlled studies of conventional antipsychotics (54–56) and novel antipsychotics (56–58) supports the modest effectiveness of these agents for the treatment of agitation and dementia compared with placebo. However, aggregate analyses of multiple trials of antipsychotics are less conclusive.

As shown in Table 4 (25,34–36,48,49, 59–65), evidence-based reviews of pharmacological treatments generally have found that antipsychotic agents are effective in the treatment of behavioral symptoms; however, meta-analyses of studies of single agents or classes of antipsychotics have shown no effect or modest improvement. In contrast, consensus statements widely support the use of antipsychotics and favor the use of novel antipsychotics over conventional agents (48,49). In addition, there is accumulating evidence that antidepressants and anticonvulsants are effective in reducing agitation and other behavioral symptoms of dementia (64).

A limited body of literature suggests that the use of cholinesterase inhibitors can result in changes in behavior and functioning that are detected by both physicians and caregivers, although these findings are based on subanalyses of trials that did not enroll patients with dementia specifically for behavioral problems (34). In addition, a considerably smaller literature base has examined treatments for depression in dementia. The effectiveness of tricyclic antidepressants for depression in dementia is not supported (66). However, a recent review suggests that SSRIs may have some benefit (34).

Behavioral and environmental modifications are also effective in enhancing functioning and reducing problem behaviors associated with dementia. Interventions include light exercise or music (34,35,67), behavioral or social reinforcement, and environmental modifications, such as access to an outdoor area, simulated home environments, and reduced-stimulation units for agitated residents (25,67). Psychoeducational training and support groups for caregivers have been shown to delay placement in nursing homes and to decrease caregiver stress (34).

In summary, empirical evidence supports the value of psychosocial interventions in addressing behavioral symptoms of dementia, but there is less agreement on the effectiveness of antipsychotic, anticonvulsant, and antidepressant agents. However, aggregate analyses of the literature should be interpreted with caution because of the substantial heterogeneity in diagnostic criteria, the inclusion of patients with different types of dementia, the variability in specification of the interventions, and the difficulty of rigorously assessing outcomes in this population.

Finally, it is imperative that clinical assessment of all behavioral and cognitive symptoms includes the differential diagnosis of delirium. The increased risk of delirium among older persons (68) and the poor prognosis (69) warrant a careful and systematic assessment of the wide spectrum of possible etiologies and the appropriate treatment of the cause and associated symptoms (70,71).

Alcohol abuse

Consensus statements (72,73) and general reviews (74,75) provide little endorsement for the effectiveness of pharmacological interventions for geriatric alcohol abuse. In contrast, psychosocial interventions are likely to be effective for older persons with alcohol use disorders (Table 5). Promising treatment components include separate treatment groups for older persons, supportive and nonconfrontational treatment approaches, and group or individual cognitive-behavioral therapy (25). In particular, there is compelling evidence that brief cognitive-behavioral interventions are effective in treating late-life alcohol abuse (76).

In summary, age-specific, nonconfrontational, brief motivational, and cognitive-behavioral therapies show promise as interventions for alcohol abuse in geriatric populations.

Schizophrenia

We found no evidence-based reviews or meta-analyses of treatment for schizophrenia among older persons. Nonetheless, a consensus statement on late-life schizophrenia (77) and general reviews of the treatment of psychosis in the elderly population (78,79) endorsed the view that antipsychotic medications are effective.

For example, reviews have compared the relative merits and potential complications of conventional antipsychotic agents (80,81) and novel antipsychotics (80–84) for the treatment of psychosis among older persons. Clinical reviews have reported that older persons are more susceptible to adverse effects of conventional antipsychotics, including parkinsonian side effects and tardive dyskinesia (80–82). Recent research on the use of novel antipsychotics among older adults is largely limited to open-label uncontrolled studies (85–88) and a small number of controlled trials (89,90). Overall, the reports and reviews suggest that atypical antipsychotics should be considered as first-line agents in the treatment of schizophrenia among older persons. Recent systematic reviews comparing the effectiveness and cost-effectiveness of conventional agents and atypical agents other than clozapine among younger patients did not find evidence of significant differences in efficacy (91,92). However, atypical agents have been shown to be safer for older persons in terms of motor side effects, especially tardive dyskinesia (93).

Data on psychosocial interventions for older adults with schizophrenia are lacking. The literature on the effectiveness of psychosocial treatments for geriatric schizophrenia is limited to a single controlled pilot study suggesting the potential benefits of a combination of cognitive-behavioral therapy and skills training (94). A consensus statement supports residential alternatives rather than long-term hospitalization and the provision of social and vocational skills training, community support programs, and psychoeducational programs for family members (77). However, the lack of data supporting these recommendations is noted, which underscores recommendations for studies addressing this research gap (1).

In summary, the efficacy of antipsychotic treatment of schizophrenia among older persons is supported by individual studies and general reviews; however, no evidence-based reviews or meta-analyses have been published.

Anxiety disorders

Anxiety is one of the most common mental health problems affecting older adults (2). However, there is a paucity of research on the effectiveness of available treatments. General reviews of the literature provide a limited perspective on the effectiveness of treatments for geriatric anxiety disorders (2,95–98). These reviews report that benzodiazepines are the most frequently prescribed antianxiety medication among older persons and recommend consideration of pharmacological alternatives. However, few double-blind placebo-controlled trials have been conducted with this population (96).

Despite preliminary results suggesting possible benefits of cognitive-behavioral therapy in the treatment of geriatric anxiety disorders, conclusive findings are not available (25,96,99).

Other promising but inadequately researched psychotherapy treatments include cognitive-behavioral group therapy, cognitive restructuring, individual behavioral therapy, and supportive group psychotherapy (2).

In summary, the limited empirical evidence confirms the efficacy of treatment with conventional antianxiety agents, while acknowledging the potential problems associated with benzodiazepines. Cognitive-behavioral therapy has the greatest support among psychosocial interventions.

Models of service delivery

In addition to research on treatments for specific disorders, a limited body of literature has examined the effectiveness of various models of service delivery. A review of the evidence base found the greatest support for community-based, multidisciplinary, geriatric mental health treatment teams (100). Promising although inconclusive data were found on the effectiveness of hospital-based geriatric psychiatry consultation-liaison services. In contrast, no randomized controlled studies have examined the effectiveness of geropsychiatric inpatient units or day hospital programs. Finally, the effectiveness of geriatric consultation services to nursing homes is inconclusive. One review (101) found a randomized controlled trial that showed no significant differences in clinical outcomes between patients who received psychiatry consultation services and those who received usual care.

In summary, empirical evidence supports the effectiveness of community-based, multidisciplinary geriatric mental health treatment teams.

Implementing evidence-based practices
Challenges
Despite evidence supporting the efficacy of a variety of interventions for geriatric mental disorders, the implementation of these interventions in usual care settings is limited. Reasons for this limited implementation include organizational barriers, bias and ageism among providers, inadequate and discriminatory financing of mental health services for older persons, and lack of collaboration and co-

ordination between providers (2,3). These barriers are further complicated by national shortages of medical and social service professionals who have training and expertise in geriatric mental health care (1,3). The different priorities, capacities, and levels of expertise between primary care, long-term care, and specialty mental health providers in the areas of aging and mental health care further complicate implementation of evidence-based treatments (3,102).

In summary, there is a substantial shortfall in the provision of psychiatric interventions in usual-care settings. Nearly half of older adults with a recognized mental disorder have unmet needs for services (103).

Implementation research
An evolving practice research literature describes methods that may effectively improve the implementation and use of evidence-based practices by mental health providers who serve older adults in usual care settings.

Primary care. Most older persons who receive mental health care are treated by primary care physicians (102,103). Yet the many demands of primary care present substantial challenges to such care (2). Older persons with psychiatric illnesses are more likely to receive inappropriate pharmacological treatment and less likely to be treated with psychotherapeutic interventions than younger primary care patients (104).

Considerable attention has been focused on educational efforts to improve screening for and treatment of depression by primary care providers, yet the failures of these traditional approaches as a means of improving physicians' practices are well documented. For example, providing practice guidelines to clinicians without additional incentives or interventions aimed at changing practices is ineffective in changing their behavior (105–107). Although physician education is necessary, it alone is not effective in enhancing guideline-concordant care. Grand rounds presentations and physician conferences, the mainstay of conventional continuing medical education, are generally ineffective by themselves (108). Educational interventions that actively involve the learner and use multiple techniques are most effective in changing physicians' behavior (106).

For example, academic detailing, which consists of brief one-on-one educational sessions coupled with provider-specific feedback on treatment practices, is effective in influencing the practice behavior of primary care physicians (109). Changes resulting from this novel educational intervention include short-term improvement in rates of detection of the target disorder (110) and a decrease in prescriptions for medications that are not indicated (109).

Other effective interventions include changing the process of care within a physician's office. For example, interventions to change the system have been found to result in significant improvements in quality of care and patient outcomes (107). Such interventions include combinations of physician and patient education, care management, and improved coordination among mental health and primary care providers. Simple but effective interventions for facilitating the process of care also include tools that monitor patients' progress, such as severity measures (111) and systems for scheduling routine follow-up visits (112). Care management can also help improve treatment adherence and facilitate monitoring of treatment response. In this model, the geriatric psychiatrist or other specialist supervises care managers and provides limited consultation to the primary care or general psychiatrist providers.

Finally, another approach is integration of services through collaboration between providers of specialty mental health care and primary care in a common setting. A mental health clinician who provides collaborative care is situated in the primary care practice setting and coordinates assessment and treatment services with the medical provider (113).

Long-term care. Observational studies suggest that mental health consultation services in nursing homes may be associated with better outcomes for residents (101). However, few randomized controlled studies of these programs have been conducted. Training in assessment and management of behavioral problems has been shown to reduce turnover of clinical staff (114) and improve the knowledge and performance of nursing staff (115,116). Educational outreach interventions are also effective in changing the clinical practice behavior of prescribing physicians when education and feedback is provided on an individual basis (117). In addition to evidence-based interventions, a series of guidelines specific to the treatment of major mental health disorders have been developed to assist nursing home professionals in caring for older adults with mental illness (118,119).

Specialty services in the community. There are few data on improving the adherence of community-based specialty mental health providers to empirically based geriatric mental health practices. General mental health clinicians lack training in basic assessment and treatment of the mental disorders of aging. System change interventions that support clinicians in the use of assessment and treatment planning toolkits have been shown to improve clinicians' adherence to standardized geriatric assessment practices (120). However, data are lacking on interventions aimed at improving the use of evidence-based treatments in community settings.

Strategies

The gap between research findings on empirically supported treatments and clinical practice suggests the need for an organized strategy to facilitate the implementation of geriatric evidence-based practices in usual care settings. Key elements of an approach to implementing evidence-based practices emphasize the involvement of stakeholder groups, including administrators, clinicians, consumers, and families (121). Implementation guides for mental health authorities and administrators are designed to address the reorganization of practice environments, procedures, incentives, and reimbursements to incorporate empirically supported treatment practices. In contrast, materials for clinicians are designed to accommodate different levels of expertise and to provide decision support technologies and treatment guides that facilitate the use of evidence-based

treatments in routine practice. Finally, the adoption of empirically supported treatments depends on buy-in by consumers and their families, who will ultimately decide to follow or reject recommended treatments. Multimedia educational materials that are sensitive to the preferences and needs of consumers and their family are important in supporting the acceptance and use of evidence-based treatments.

In summary, a successful strategy for implementing evidence-based mental health interventions is grounded in a systems approach, combined with the development and dissemination of easy-to-use implementation kits and well-described procedures for changing practices (121).

Conclusions

This overview of research defining evidence-based practices in geriatric mental health care suggests that there is a need to address the profound gap between research findings on effective treatments and the current availability of such treatments for older persons with mental disorders.

However, several caveats are indicated in considering such an effort. First, identification of evidence-based practices should be considered as a starting point for improving the quality of care. In essence, evidence-based practices define "the floor" in quality and should not be confused with best, optimal, or promising practices. Second, there is a misperception that only randomized controlled trials, meta-analyses, or systematic reviews can constitute the evidence base. Evidence-based practice is based on careful and appropriate use of the findings of the best relevant studies, accompanied by an appreciation of the limits of the existing data. In some instances, the best studies include randomized controlled trials, whereas in other situations, nonrandomized outcome studies or case reports may constitute the evidence base.

An additional and important consideration involves inherent limitations in the methodology used to identify evidence-based practices, which may result in the overly conservative exclusion of informative studies or may group studies together without adequate attention to important differ-

ences between studies. For example, common problems affecting meta-analyses and evidence-based reviews include small samples and lack of power, heterogeneity of samples, lack of interchangeable instruments, lack of extractable data, different definitions of outcomes, differences in the quality of research and the duration of the studies, and reliance on statistical rather than clinical significance (63,122).

Furthermore, evidence-based reviews and meta-analyses are largely dependent on data from randomized controlled trials that compare a single well-defined intervention with a placebo or other control. Thus they are less suited to inform more complex decisions, such as choosing the next step after a series of failed interventions for a treatment-refractory condition or making the most effective use of the many different possible combinations of agents. The large number of potential combinations and sequences of treatments and the large number of different clinical conditions and comorbid physical conditions make it virtually impossible to support all clinical decisions with data from randomized controlled trials (8).

One approach to addressing gaps left by standardized evidence-based reviews and meta-analyses is the use of expert consensus guidelines. Recently published guidelines on the pharmacotherapy of depression among older patients are an example of treatment recommendations based on an aggregate analysis of independent ratings by experts on the appropriateness of various treatment options (18). In addition, the guidelines for major psychiatric disorders developed by the American Psychiatric Association (APA) (36,70, 123–127) provide treatment recommendations that are assigned one of three levels of confidence based on clinical consensus. With the exception of the guidelines on dementia, the APA guidelines are not age specific, suggesting that future initiatives may be undertaken to develop clinical guidelines specific to older adults.

In general, guidelines and treatment algorithms can provide the clinician with a practical and comprehensive summary of recommendations. However, caution is warranted.

Guidelines should be evaluated on the basis of their level of support from systematic reviews of the evidence, because the consensus of experts may inadvertently incorporate the bias of specialties and disciplines and may misrepresent treatment effectiveness or side effects (128,129).

Finally, despite advances in clinical expertise and research, a substantial body of literature chronicles the failure of conventional educational approaches and the limited impact of disseminating treatment guidelines. Meaningful changes in the quality of care require innovative technologies that use research findings focused on organizational and provider change. This challenge is compounded in a system of geriatric mental health care that includes different organizations and sources of financing and treatment by providers from different disciplines. Despite these challenges, there is a clear and urgent demographic imperative to address the emerging public health problem of the mental disorders of aging. It is time for geriatric psychiatry to take up the mantle of evidence-based practices and translate research findings into the mainstream of clinical treatment for older Americans. ◆

References

1. Jeste DV, Alexopoulos GS, Bartels SJ, et al: Consensus statement on the upcoming crisis in geriatric mental health: research agenda for the next two decades. Archives of General Psychiatry 56:848–853, 1999

2. Mental Health: A Report of the Surgeon General. Rockville, Md, US Department of Health and Human Services, 1999

3. Older Adults and Mental Health: Issues and Opportunities. Rockville, Md, Administration on Aging, US Department of Health and Human Services, 2001

4. Bartels SJ: Quality, costs, and effectiveness of services for older adults with mental disorders: a selective overview of recent advances in geriatric mental health services research. Current Opinion in Psychiatry 15: 411–416, 2002

5. Institute of Medicine: Crossing the Quality Chasm: A New Health System for the 21st Century. Washington, DC, National Academy Press, 2001

6. Bridging Science and Service. Rockville, Md, National Institute of Mental Health, 1999

7. Cochrane AL: Effectiveness and Efficiency: Random Reflections on Health Services. London, Nuffield Provincial Hospitals Trust, 1972

8. Guyatt G, Rennie D: Users' Guide to the Medical Literature: A Manual for Evidence-Based Clinical Practice. Chicago, Evidence-Based Medicine Working Group American Medical Association, AMA Press, 2002

9. Sackett DL, Rosenberg WM, Gray JA, et al: Evidence-based medicine: what it is and what it isn't. British Medical Journal 312: 71–72, 1996

10. Robins LN, Regier DA: Psychiatric Disorders in America: The Epidemiologic Catchment Area Study. New York, Free Press, 1991

11. Thorpe L, Whitney DK, Kutcher SP, et al: Clinical guidelines for the treatment of depressive disorders: VI. special populations. Canadian Journal of Psychiatry 46:63S–76S, 2001

12. Wilson K, Mottram P, Sivanranthan A, et al: Antidepressant versus placebo for depressed elderly (Cochrane Review) in Cochrane Library. Oxford, England, Update Software, 2001

13. Anderson IM: Selective serotonin reuptake inhibitors versus tricyclic antidepressants: a meta-analysis of efficacy and tolerability. Journal of Affective Disorders 58:19–36, 2000

14. Gerson S, Belin TR, Kaufman A, et al: Pharmacological and psychological treatments for depressed older patients: a meta-analysis and overview of recent findings. Harvard Review of Psychiatry 7:1–28, 1999

15. Mulrow CD, Williams JW, Trivedi M, et al: Treatment of Depression: Newer Pharmacotherapies. Evidence Report, Technology Assessment 7. AHCPR pub no 99-E014. Rockville, Md, Agency for Health Care Policy and Research, 1999

16. McCusker J, Cole M, Keller E, et al: Effectiveness of treatments of depression in older ambulatory patients. Archives of Internal Medicine 158:705–712, 1998

17. Mittmann N, Herrmann N, Einarson TR, et al: The efficacy, safety, and tolerability of antidepressants in late life depression: a meta-analysis. Journal of Affective Disorders 46:191–217, 1997

18. Alexopoulos GS, Katz IR, Reynolds CF, et al: The Expert Consensus Guideline Series: pharmacotherapy of depressive disorders in older patients. Postgraduate Medicine 110 (Oct special report):1–86, 2001

19. Mulsant BH, Alexopoulos GS, Reynolds CF III, et al: Pharmacological treatment of depression in older primary care patients: the PROSPECT algorithm. International Journal of Geriatric Psychiatry 16:585–592, 2001

20. American Society of Health-System Pharmacists: Therapeutic position statement on the recognition and treatment of depression in older adults. American Journal of Health-System Pharmacy 55:2514–2518, 1998

21. Lebowitz BD, Pearson JL, Schneider LS, et al: Diagnosis and treatment of depression in late life: consensus statement update. JAMA 278:1186–1190, 1997

22. NIH consensus development conference statement: diagnosis and treatment of depression in late life. JAMA 268:1018–1024, 1992

23. Kirsch I, Moore TJ, Scoboria A, et al: The em tamine for the Treatment of Alzheimer's Disease. Technology Appraisal Guidance no 19. National Institute for Clinical Excellence, London, 2001

38. Birks J, Flicker L: Selegiline for Alzheimer's disease (Cochrane Review) in Cochrane Library. Oxford, England, Update Software, 2001

39. Birks JS, Melzer D, Beppu H: Donepezil for mild and moderate Alzheimer's disease (Cochrane Review) in Cochrane Library. Oxford, England, Update Software, 2001

40. Fioravanti M, Flicker L: Efficacy of nicergoline in dementia and other age associated forms of cognitive impairment (Cochrane Review) in Cochrane Library. Oxford, England, Update Software, 2001

41. Fioravanti M, Yanagi M: Cytidinediphosphocholine (CDP choline) for cognitive and behavioral disturbances associated with chronic cerebral disorders in the elderly (Cochrane Review) in Cochrane Library. Oxford, England, Update Software, 2001

42. Olin J, Schneider L: Galantamine for Alzheimer's disease (Cochrane Review) in Cochrane Library. Oxford, England, Update Software, 2001

43. Spector A, Orrell M, Davies S, et al: Reality orientation for dementia (Cochrane Review) in Cochrane Library. Oxford, England, Update Software, 2001

44. Birks J, Grimley EJ, Iakovidou V, et al: Rivastigmine for Alzheimer's disease (Cochrane Review) in Cochrane Library. Oxford, England, Update Software, 2000

45. Higgins JPT, Flicker L: Lecithin for dementia and cognitive impairment (Cochrane Review) in Cochrane Library. Oxford, England, Update Software, 2000

46. Qizilbash N, Whitehead A, Higgins J, et al: Cholinesterase inhibition for Alzheimer disease: a meta-analysis of the tacrine trials. JAMA 280:1777–1782, 1998

47. Oken BS, Storzbach DM, Kaye JA: The efficacy of ginkgo biloba on cognitive function in Alzheimer disease. Archives of Neurology 55:1409–1415, 1998

48. Patterson CJ, Gauthier S, Bergman H, et al: The recognition, assessment, and management of dementing disorders: conclusions from the Canadian Consensus Conference on Dementia. Canadian Medical Association Journal 160(12 suppl):S1–15, 1999

49. Small GW, Rabins PV, Barry PP, et al: Diagnosis and treatment of Alzheimer disease and related disorders: consensus statement of the American Association for Geriatric Psychiatry, the Alzheimer's Association, and the American Geriatrics Society. JAMA 278:1363–1371, 1997

50. Lopez OL, Becker JT, Wisniewski S, et al: Cholinesterase inhibitor treatment alters the natural history of Alzheimer's disease. Journal of Neurology and Neurosurgical Psychiatry 72:310–314, 2002

51. Feldman H, Gauthier S, Hecker J, et al: A

24-week, randomized, double-blind study of donepezil in moderate to severe Alzheimer's disease. Neurology 57:613–620, 2001

52. Erkinjuntti T, Kurz A, Gauthier S, et al: Efficacy of galantamine in probable vascular dementia and Alzheimer's disease combined with cerebrovascular disease: a randomised trial. Lancet 359:1283–1290, 2002

53. Tabet N, Birks J, Grimley Evans J, et al: Vitamin E for Alzheimer's disease (Cochrane Review) in Cochrane Library. Oxford, England, Update Software, 2001

54. Devanand DP, Marder K, Michaels KS, et al: A randomized, placebo-controlled dose-comparison trial of haloperidol for psychosis and disruptive behaviors in Alzheimer's disease. American Journal of Psychiatry 155:1512–1520, 1998

55. Teri L, Logsdon RG, Peskind E, et al: Treatment of agitation in Alzheimer's disease: a randomized, placebo-controlled clinical trial. Neurology 55:1271–1278, 2000

56. De Deyn P, Rabheru K, Rasmussen A, et al: A randomized trial of risperidone, placebo, and haloperidol for behavioral symptoms of dementia. Neurology 53:946–955, 1999

57. Katz IR, Jeste DV, Mintzer JE, et al: Comparison of risperidone and placebo for psychosis and behavioral disturbances associated with dementia: a randomized, double-blind trial. Journal of Clinical Psychiatry 60:107–115, 1999

58. Bhana N, Spencer CM: Risperidone: a review of its use in the management of the behavioural and psychological symptoms of dementia. Drugs and Aging 16:451–471, 2000

59. Kirchner V, Kelley CA, Harvey RJ: Thioridazine for dementia (Cochrane Review) in Cochrane Library. Oxford, England, Update Software, 2001

60. Lonergan E, Luxenberg J, Colford J: Haloperidol for agitation in dementia (Cochrane Review) in Cochrane Library. Oxford, England, Update Software, 2001

61. Olin J, Schneider L, Novit A, et al: Hydergine for dementia (Cochrane Review) in Cochrane Library. Oxford, England, Update Software, 2001

62. Lanctot KL, Best TS, Mittmann N, et al: Efficacy and safety of neuroleptics in behavioral disorders associated with dementia. Journal of Clinical Psychiatry 59:550–561, 1998

63. Schneider LS, Pollock VE, Lyness SA: A meta-analysis of controlled trials of neuroleptic treatment in dementia. Journal of the American Geriatrics Society 38:553–563, 1990

64. Herrmann N: Recommendations for the management of behavioral and psychological symptoms of dementia. Canadian Journal of Neurological Sciences 28(suppl 1):S96–S107, 2001

65. Alexopoulos GS, Silver JM, Kahn DA, et al: The expert consensus guideline series: treatment of agitation in older persons with dementia. Postgraduate Medicine 104(Apr special report):1–88, 1998

66. Mayeux R, Sano M: Treatment of Alzheimer's disease. New England Journal of Medicine 341:1670–1679, 1999

67. Cohen-Mansfield J: Nonpharmacologic interventions for inappropriate behaviors in dementia. American Journal of Geriatric Psychiatry 9:361–381, 2001

68. Elie M, Cole MG, Primeau FJ, et al: Delirium risk factors in elderly hospitalized patients. Journal of General Internal Medicine 13:204–12, 1998

69. Cole MG, Primeau FJ: Prognosis of delirium in elderly hospital patients. Canadian Medical Association Journal 149:41–46, 1993

70. American Psychiatric Association: Practice guideline for the treatment of patients with delirium. American Journal of Psychiatry 156(5 suppl):1–20, 1999

71. Cole MG, Primeau FJ, Elie LM: Delirium: prevention, treatment, and outcome studies. Journal of Geriatric Psychiatry and Neurology 11:126–137, 1998

72. Substance Abuse Among Older Adults. Treatment Improvement Protocol, 26. Rockville, Md, Center for Substance Abuse Treatment, 1998

73. Council on Scientific Affairs of the American Medical Association: Alcoholism in the elderly. JAMA 275:797–801, 1996

74. Schonfeld L, Dupree LW: Treatment approaches for older problem drinkers. International Journal of the Addictions 30:1819–1842, 1995

75. Fingerhood M: Substance abuse in older people. Journal of the American Geriatrics Society 48:985–995, 2000

76. Blow FC, Barry KL: Older patients with at-risk and problem drinking patterns: new developments in brief interventions. Journal of Geriatric Psychiatry and Neurology 13:115–123, 2000

77. Cohen CI, Cohen GD, Blank K, et al: Schizophrenia and older adults: an overview: directions for research and policy. American Journal of Geriatric Psychiatry 8:19–28, 2000

78. Soares JC, Gershon S: Therapeutic targets in late-life psychoses: review of concepts and critical issues. Schizophrenia Research 27:227–239, 1997

79. Lake JT, Rahman AH, Grossberg GT: Diagnosis and treatment of psychotic symptoms in elderly patients. Drugs and Aging 11:170–177, 1997

80. Maixner SM, Mellow AM, Tandon R: The efficacy, safety, and tolerability of antipsychotics in the elderly. Journal of Clinical Psychiatry 60:29–41, 1999

81. Finkel SI: Antipsychotics: old and new. Clinics in Geriatric Medicine 14:87–100, 1998

82. Chan YC, Pariser SF, Neufeld G: Atypical antipsychotics in older adults. Pharmacotherapy 19:811–822, 1999

83. Kumar V: Use of atypical antipsychotic agents in geriatric patients: a review. International Journal of Geriatric Psychopharmacology 1:15–23, 1997

84. Sweet RA, Pollock BG: New atypical antipsychotics: experience and utility in the elderly. Drugs and Aging 12:115–127, 1998

85. Davidson M, Harvey PD, Vervarcke J, et al: A long-term, multicenter, open-label study of risperidone in elderly patients with psychosis. International Journal of Geriatric Psychiatry 15:506–514, 2000

86. Tariot PN, Salzman C, Yeung PP, et al: Long-term use of quetiapine in elderly patients with psychotic disorders. Clinical Therapeutics 22:1068–1084, 2000

87. McManus D, Arvanitis L, Kowalcyk B: Quetiapine, a novel antipsychotic: experience in elderly patients with psychotic disorders. Journal of Clinical Psychiatry 60:292–298, 1999

88. Madhusoodanan S, Brenner R, Suresh P, et al: Efficacy and tolerability of olanzapine in elderly patients with psychotic disorders: a prospective study. Annals of Clinical Psychiatry 12:11–18, 2000

89. Verma S, Orengo CA, Kunik ME, et al: Tolerability and effectiveness of atypical antipsychotics in male geriatric inpatients. International Journal of Geriatric Psychiatry 16:223–227, 2001

90. Howanitz E, Pardo M, Smelson DA, et al: The efficacy and safety of clozapine versus chlorpromazine in geriatric schizophrenia. Journal of Clinical Psychiatry 60:41–44, 1999

91. Leucht S, Pitschel-Walz G, Abraham D, et al: Efficacy and extrapyramidal side-effects of the new antipsychotics olanzapine, quetiapine, risperidone, and sertindole compared to conventional antipsychotics and placebo: a meta-analysis of randomized controlled trials. Schizophrenia Research 35:51–68, 1999

92. Geddes J, Freemantle N, Harrison P, et al: Atypical antipsychotics in the treatment of schizophrenia: systematic overview and meta-regression analysis. British Medical Journal 321:1371–1376, 2000

93. Jeste DV, Okamoto A, Napolitano J, et al: Low incidence of persistent tardive dyskinesia in elderly patients with dementia treated with risperidone. American Journal of Psychiatry 157:1150–1155, 2000

94. Granholm E, McQuaid JR, McClure FS, et al: A randomized controlled pilot study of cognitive behavioral social skills training for older patients with schizophrenia. Schizophrenia Research 53:167–169, 2002

95. Krasucki C, Howard R, Mann A: Anxiety and its treatment in the elderly. International Psychogeriatrics 11:25–45, 1999

96. Stanley MA, Beck JG: Anxiety disorders. Clinical Psychology Review 20:731–754, 2000

97. Sheikh JI, Cassidy EL: Treatment of anxiety disorders in the elderly: issues and strategies. Journal of Anxiety Disorders 14:173–190, 2000

98. Dada F, Sethi S, Grossberg GT: Generalized anxiety disorder in the elderly. Psychi-

atric Clinics of North America 24:p155–164, 2001

99. Stanley MA, Novy DM: Cognitive-behavior therapy for generalized anxiety in late life: an evaluative overview. Journal of Anxiety Disorders 14:191–207, 2000

100. Draper B: The effectiveness of old age psychiatry services. International Journal of Geriatric Psychiatry 15:687–703, 2000

101. Bartels SJ, Moak GS, Dums AR: Models of mental health services in nursing homes. Psychiatric Services 53:1390–1396, 2002

102. Burns BJ, Taube CA: Mental health services in general medical care and nursing homes, in Mental Health Policy for Older Americans: Protecting Minds at Risk. Edited by Fogel B, Furino A, Gottlieb G. Washington, DC, American Psychiatric Press, 1990

103. George LK, Blazer DG, Winfield-Laird I, et al: Psychiatric disorders and mental health service use in later life, in Epidemiology and Aging. Edited by Brody JA, Maddox GL. New York, Springer, 1988

104. Bartels SJ, Horn S, Sharkey P, et al: Treatment of depression in older primary care patients in health maintenance organizations. International Journal of Psychiatry in Medicine 27:215–231, 1997

105. Grimshaw JM, Russell IT: Effect of clinical guidelines on medical practice: a systematic review of rigorous evaluations. Lancet 342:1317–1322, 1993

106. Oxman TE: Effective educational techniques for primary care providers: application to the management of psychiatric disorders. International Journal of Psychiatry in Medicine 28:3–9, 1998

107. Callahan CM: Quality improvement research on late life depression in primary care. Medical Care 39:772–784, 2001

108. Davis DA, Thomson MA, Oxman AD, et al: Changing physician performance: a systematic review of the effect of continuing medical education strategies. JAMA 274:700–705, 1995

109. Soumerai SB: Principles and uses of academic detailing to improve the management of psychiatric disorders. International Journal of Psychiatry in Medicine 28:81–96, 1998

110. Pond C, Mant A, Kehoe L, et al: General practitioner diagnosis of depression and dementia in the elderly: can academic detailing make a difference? Family Practice 11:141–147, 1994

111. Brody D, Dietrich AJ, deGruy F: The Depression in Primary Care Tool Kit. International Journal of Psychiatry in Medicine 30:99–110, 2000

112. Lin EH, Von Korff M, Katon W, et al: The role of the primary care physician in patients' adherence to antidepressant therapy. Medical Care 33:67–74, 1995

113. Katon W, Von Korff M, Lin E, et al: Collaborative management to achieve treatment guidelines: impact on depression in primary care. JAMA 273:1026–1031, 1995

114. Sbordone RJ, Sterman LT: The psychologist as a consultant in a nursing home: effect on staff morale and turnover. Professional Psychology: Research and Practice 14:240–250, 1983

115. Smith M, Mitchell S, Buckwalter KC, et al: Geropsychiatric nursing consultation: a valuable resource in rural long term care. Archives of Psychiatric Nursing 8:272–279, 1994

116. Smyer MA, Brannon D, Cohn MD: Improving nursing home care through training and job redesign. Gerontologist 33:327–333, 1992

117. Thomson O'Brien MA, Oxman AD, Davis DA, et al: Educational outreach visits: effects on professional practice and health care outcomes (Cochrane Review) in Cochrane Library. Oxford, England, Update Software, 2001

118. Dementia. Columbia, Md, American Medical Directors Association, 1998

119. Pharmacotherapy Companion to Depression. Columbia, Md, American Medical Directors Association, 1998

120. Bartels SJ, Miles KM, Dums AR: Improving the quality of care for older adults with mental disorders: the Outcomes-Based Treatment Planning System of the New Hampshire–Dartmouth Psychiatric Research Center. The Home Care Research Initiative, Spring 2002, pp 1–6

121. Torrey WC, Drake RE, Dixon L, et al: Implementing evidence-based practices for persons with severe mental illnesses. Psychiatric Services 52:45–50, 2001

122. Schneider LS: Starving to Death in a Sea of Data: Perspectives on Translating Geriatric Psychiatry Research. Presented at the annual meeting of the American Association for Geriatric Psychiatry, Orlando, Fla, February 24–27, 2002

123. American Psychiatric Association: Practice guideline for the treatment of patients with substance use disorders: alcohol, cocaine, opioids. American Journal of Psychiatry 152(11 suppl):1–80, 1995

124. American Psychiatric Association: Practice guideline for the treatment of patients with schizophrenia. American Journal of Psychiatry 154(4 suppl):1–63, 1997

125. American Psychiatric Association: Practice guideline for the treatment of patients with panic disorder. American Journal of Psychiatry 155(5 suppl):1–34, 1998

126. American Psychiatric Association: Practice guideline for the treatment of patients with major depressive disorder (revision). American Journal of Psychiatry 157(4 suppl):1–45, 2000

127. American Psychiatric Association: Practice guideline for the treatment of patients with bipolar disorder (revision). American Journal of Psychiatry 159(4 suppl):1–50, 2002

128. Shaneyfelt TM, Mayo-Smith MF, Rothwangl J: Are guidelines following guidelines? The methodological quality of clinical practice guidelines in the peer-reviewed medical literature. JAMA 281:1900–1905, 1999

129. Grilli R, Margrini N, Penna A, et al: Practice guidelines developed by specialty societies: the need for a critical appraisal. Lancet 355:103–106, 2000

Policy Implications for Implementing Evidence-Based Practices

Howard H. Goldman, M.D., Ph.D.
Vijay Ganju, Ph.D.
Robert E. Drake, M.D., Ph.D.
Paul Gorman, Ed.D.
Michael Hogan, Ph.D.
Pamela S. Hyde, J.D.
Oscar Morgan

The authors describe the policy and administrative-practice implications of implementing evidence-based services, particularly in public-sector settings. They review the observations of the contributors to the evidence-based practices series published throughout 2001 in *Psychiatric Services*. Quality and accountability have become the watchwords of health and mental health services; evidence-based practices are a means to both ends. If the objective of accountable, high-quality services is to be achieved by implementing evidence-based practices, the right incentives must be put in place, and systemic barriers must be overcome. The authors use the framework from the U.S. Surgeon General's 1999 report on mental health to describe eight courses of action for addressing the gap between science and practice: continue to build the science base; overcome stigma; improve public awareness of effective treatments; ensure the supply of mental health services and providers; ensure delivery of state-of-the-art treatments; tailor treatment to age, sex, race, and culture; facilitate entry into treatment; and reduce financial barriers to treatment.

The U.S. Surgeon General's 1999 report on mental health (1) alerted the public, mental health advocates, and policy makers to the disparity between the opportunities for improving treatment and services and the reality of everyday practice. Services and programs based on scientific advances in treatment and services are not routinely available to meet the needs of individuals who have mental illness. The report identified

courses of action and called on the field to "ensure the supply of mental health services and providers" and "ensure delivery of state-of-the-art treatments."

Throughout 2001, each issue of *Psychiatric Services* has focused attention on this public health problem and has offered a range of responses to the Surgeon General's call to action. Various articles have reviewed individual evidence-based practices for adults and children. They have de-

scribed efforts to implement these practices, highlighting facilitators and barriers, including rules, regulations, and mental health financing policies. In this article we synthesize that material, focusing on the role of policy makers in the process of implementing evidence-based practices, particularly in the public sector.

Returning to a focus on policy and administrative practices brings us full circle in the process of reforming mental health services. In the earliest stages of the community mental health and community support reforms, emphasis was placed on organizational and financing solutions to the problems of individuals with mental illness, particularly those with severe and persistent mental disorders (2–4). Treatment technology was comparatively weak, and the reforms focused on the locus of treatment in the community and on the system of care (4).

Evaluations of several national service demonstrations have indicated that although system reforms occurred, the direct impact of system changes on individuals was limited (4–6). When system interventions alone proved necessary but insufficient for improving the lives of persons with mental illness, attention shifted to the content and quality of services. Research identified both the potential benefits of services and treatments and the deficiencies in usual care (1,7).

Both policies and administrative practices have been identified as specific barriers to the implementation of evidence-based services; policies have also been identified as facilita-

Dr. Goldman is affiliated with the department of psychiatry at the University of Maryland School of Medicine, 685 Baltimore Street, MSTF Building, Room 300, Baltimore, Maryland 21201 (e-mail, hgoldman@erols.com). Dr. Ganju is with the National Association of State Mental Health Program Directors Research Institute in Alexandria, Virginia. Dr. Drake is with Dartmouth Medical School and the New Hampshire–Dartmouth Psychiatric Research Center in Lebanon, New Hampshire. Mr. Gorman is with the West Institute for Implementing Evidence-Based Practices in Lebanon, New Hampshire. Dr. Hogan is commissioner of mental health in Ohio. Ms. Hyde is with the Technical Assistance Collaborative office in Santa Fe, New Mexico. Mr. Morgan is director of the Maryland Mental Hygiene Administration in Baltimore. This article was originally published in the December 2001 issue of Psychiatric Services.

tors. Policies create incentives and disincentives that shape the mental health service system. A major challenge is to identify policy interventions that facilitate implementation of evidence- based practices but also minimize barriers to implementation. This article is addressed to policy makers and to those who advise them and who would influence their rules and regulations—namely, the rest of us.

Quality and accountability

Quality and accountability have become the watchwords of health and mental health services (8). Implementing evidence-based practices has become a means to achieving both ends. In this context "quality" means positive outcomes obtained by using cost-effective services, and "accountability" means documentation of adherence to evidence-based practice.

Michael Hogan, commissioner of mental health in Ohio, refers to a triangular relationship among these three service system elements: quality improvement, accountability through performance measurement, and evidence-based practices. He describes this relationship as central to providing effective mental health services (personal communication, Hogan M, 2001). Implementing evidence-based practices is a quality-improvement process that provides accountability through the monitoring of the fidelity of practices to models that have been demonstrated by research to be effective.

Using this framework, policy makers can approach their funders with greater confidence. They can argue for resources to implement evidence-based practices with greater assurance of accountability and value for money. Monitoring for adherence to evidence-based practices is possible through the use of fidelity measures. Programs that are faithful to the evidence-based models produce good outcomes in general, but not necessarily for all individuals or for all circumstances. Achieving consistently positive outcomes is at the heart of the definition of an evidence-based practice.

With common agreement about the validity and appropriateness of these positive outcomes as policy goals, the quality of mental health services can be continually improved. Measures of

fidelity, like other process measures, are a means to an end, not an end in themselves. It is critical that fidelity to a particular model or practice not be regulated in a way that prevents client choice, clinical judgment, or continuing change as new evidence emerges. Yet fidelity should be a goal to which systems and practitioners aspire, with the assumption that the greater the fidelity, the greater the likelihood of good outcomes.

Unfortunately, although the Surgeon General concluded that a range

A major challenge is to identify policy interventions that facilitate implementation of evidence-based practices but also minimize barriers to implementation.

of efficacious treatments exists for almost every mental disorder, for many clinical conditions there is no evidence to support particular treatments or services. For example, although effective treatments are available for schizophrenia and bipolar disorders, many patients with these disorders have complications and comorbid disorders that have not been considered in studies of treatment effectiveness. In many cases, the existing evidence comes from clinical trials that may not be generalizable without adaptation to typical treatment settings—for example, the trials may have been conducted by clinicians with specific levels of training or with homogeneous patient groups.

For some problems with the greatest salience—such as youth suicide, posttraumatic stress disorder, and

borderline personality disorder—there is not yet a satisfactory research base to guide policy and practice with clarity, although the evidence base for each of these problems is growing. Rosenberg and colleagues (9) have suggested that while we wait for definitive answers to emerge, policy makers hold off on endorsing specific models and instead support studies of comparative effectiveness.

Not every problem has an evidence-based solution, and not every evidence-based practice that works for a majority of persons who have similar symptoms, history, and needs will work for all such individuals. There continues to be much room for clinical judgment, client choice, and development of innovative treatments and services. However, evidence-based practices do exist for certain clinical conditions, as documented in the pages of this journal throughout the past year. Yet too often these practices are not implemented, even when their benefits are well understood; when clients, clinicians, and policy makers agree on desired outcomes; or when models exist of successful implementation.

States are moving forward in their implementation of evidence-based practices with varying levels of commitment and success. Many are struggling with the implementation of evidence-based practices that have existed for more than a decade and that have been proven effective in a variety of settings. Even when states have had the political and administrative will—or at least the stated interest—to implement evidence-based practices, they have not always done so by using mechanisms that ensure adherence to fidelity. And even when evidence-based services have been implemented with fidelity, systems have had to address questions of how these fit with each other and with services that lack a strong evidence base.

Many factors contribute to these implementation problems, including lack of a long-term vision for the service system, lack of agreement on desired outcomes, lack of penalties for practices that are not evidence based, short-term horizons for policy planning, political mandates or competing public-sector priorities, resource limitations, and uncertainty associated with change and untoward events. In such a context, administrative practice and the policy infrastructure are of paramount importance.

Overcoming systemic barriers

Although the focus has shifted from organization and financing to the content and quality of services, policy makers cannot ignore the systemic barriers to implementing evidence-based practices. Each of the articles on evidence-based practices has identified barriers related to organizational policy and financing policy, and some have identified strategies for overcoming those barriers and creating appropriate incentives to support implementation. We use the eight courses of action outlined by the Surgeon General to organize this section.

Continue to build the science base

As we have noted, there are limitations in the treatment-effectiveness research base that defines the evidence-based practices. More research is needed to determine whether these practices are effective in all ethnic subpopulations, among persons who have multiple disorders, and in all practice settings—for example, rural as opposed to urban settings. In addition, more research is needed on nontraditional approaches that give clients more control of their own recovery or that utilize professionals trained in nontraditional methods.

Furthermore, although thousands of studies have been conducted on dissemination of innovation and implementation of health and mental health services, there is virtually no definitive evidence to guide implementation of specific evidence-based practices. However, some experts, such as Argyris (10), warn that the results of experimental studies that involve human interaction may not generalize to any great degree to typical treatment circumstances, because the complexity of social systems cannot be captured in controlled experiments. There is uncomfortable irony in moving forward to implement evidence-based practices in the absence of an evidence base to guide implementation practice.

Torrey and colleagues (7) reviewed some of the literature on dissemination and implementation but uncovered more about what we do not know than about what we do know. The literature is better at telling us what does not work and what not to do than it is at guiding our work. We intend to study the earliest experiences with evidence-based practices to identify significant barriers and successful strategies to inform future implementation efforts.

More research is needed to determine whether these practices are effective in all ethnic subpopulations, among persons who have multiple disorders, and in all practice settings.

Overcome stigma

Few of the authors in the evidence-based practices series in *Psychiatric Services* identified stigma as a special barrier to implementing evidence-based practices. However, a special section of four research articles in this issue of the journal examines stigma as a barrier to recovery. It is possible that the pervasive stigma associated with mental illness and its treatment has resulted in discriminatory financing policies. As a result of stigma, individuals who are in need are unwilling to seek care. They experience forms of discrimination that can exacerbate their illness if they do seek treatment. In addition, stigma often produces service delivery systems that view mental health treatment as less valuable or

necessary than general health care.

For example, all too often Medicaid does not cover the evidence-based practices or covers them in a way that precludes faithful implementation of the model. With lack of fidelity comes the risk of losing the positive outcomes documented in the research. Furthermore, there is growing evidence that budgets for public mental health systems are eroding (11). All the authors in the evidence-based practices series identified financing policies as barriers to implementing evidence-based practices.

Improve public awareness of effective treatments

All the articles began with a careful description of evidence-based practices. It cannot be assumed that all readers of *Psychiatric Services* are familiar with all the evidence-based practices, let alone understand all the barriers to and facilitators of implementation. Although awareness alone is not sufficient for implementation, it is certainly a necessary first step. Consumers and family members can affect the demand for evidence-based services if they are aware of the benefits associated with these services (12). Evidence from general medical care supports the effectiveness of raising awareness (13). Providers—both clinicians and administrators—must understand the new practices and their utility before they can be expected to adopt them. The same, of course, is true for policy makers.

Ensure the supply of mental health services and providers

Ensuring the supply of mental health services and providers, along with the next course of action—ensuring the delivery of state-of-the-art treatments—is at the heart of the matter. Policy makers have a responsibility to ensure that individual clinicians and service providers are available in their mental health systems. This responsibility involves making a commitment to recruiting individuals who have the necessary skills to deliver evidence-based services, creating incentives to attract these individuals to practice in their systems, and training, supervising, and supporting the work of providers of evidence-based services.

Retaining skilled providers and minimizing job burnout are critical to maintaining a workforce that is capable of supplying evidence-based services. According to the Surgeon General and the authors of the articles in the *Psychiatric Services* evidence-based practices series, there is a shortage of trained personnel who are able to provide the evidence-based services described. The erosion of the resources of state mental health programs undermines the ability of mental health agencies to attract and retain competent clinicians. It will be necessary to develop mechanisms for retraining the current workforce and to influence the training of new professionals and paraprofessionals.

The Evidence-Based Practices Project, which is described in more detail below, is designed to increase the number of individuals and clinical service teams who are able to practice in a manner that is supported by research findings. Some practices require that consumer-providers and family members receive special training. All need informed and engaged individuals at all levels of service provision—consumers, family members, clinicians, program administrators, and policy makers.

Without these informed and committed administrators and policy makers, no amount of literature or evidence will matter, and no amount of accountability through measurement of fidelity will increase public commitment to seeking or funding mental health care. Fidelity will give way to whatever clinicians can get paid for, and accountability will give way to whatever questions funders want answered. Program administrators need assistance in understanding the need, making the case, and sustaining the effort to lead systems either to promote evidence-based practices or, at least, to get out of the way.

Ensure delivery of state-of-the-art treatments

Each of the authors of the papers on evidence-based practices reinforced the need for leadership in implementing state-of-the-art practices. The authors also pointed out that ensuring delivery is not a trivial matter. Evidence-based practices must be a

priority for care. Architects of the mental health system must organize services with quality improvement in mind. Regulations often impede the implementation of evidence-based practices. It is not possible to deliver state-of-the-art treatments if, for example, newer antipsychotic medications are not on the formulary of a program, or if an insurer does not cover family interventions.

Regulations may create unanticipated barriers. For example, supported employment may not be an approved service for Medicaid reim-

The Surgeon General encouraged multiple "portals of entry" to mental health services by creating incentives for many service providers to receive referrals and accept all individuals seeking services.

bursement. Most states cannot afford to offer evidence-based services without Medicaid coverage; often, a majority of individuals in public-sector programs are not eligible for Medicaid. Organizational and financial barriers to integrated treatment have been identified for supported employment (between vocational rehabilitation and mental health agencies) and for integrated treatment of co-occurring substance abuse and severe mental illness (between separate substance abuse and mental health service authorities). This is a special problem in which federal mental health

and substance abuse block grant funds cannot be mingled to provide integrated care. Overcoming these agencies' divisions is often an important first step in the effort to provide better-integrated services. On the other hand, some of these services, such as assertive community treatment, are designed to provide the services themselves instead of relying on a fragmented service system.

Tailor treatment to age, sex, race, and culture

Although the research base is not sufficient to support all the evidence-based practices with each of the sociodemographic groups encountered in practice, it is always important to be culturally sensitive and respectful of diversity when designing and delivering services. It is also important to realize that, for the most part, when research on evidence-based practices has been conducted in ethnic subpopulations, the outcomes have been good. As emphasized by the Surgeon General, tailoring treatment will be of special importance in situations in which "culture counts" in specific ways (14).

For example, family interventions must take into account the cultural meanings of family and respect the differences in meaning associated with age, sex, and stage of the life cycle. Language-appropriate services are critical to successful outreach and for encouraging members of linguistic minorities to use evidence-based services. Medications should be used appropriately, with an awareness of ethnopsychopharmacologic variations in physiology and in attitudes and behaviors associated with drug taking. In addition to being faithful to program models, evidence-based services must reach out and include everyone in a community who might need or benefit from the services.

Facilitate entry into treatment

In most cases, people cannot benefit from evidence-based treatments if they do not seek help. Occasionally treatment is provided under a court order, but in general the goal is to have consumers receive services on a voluntary basis. Evidence-based services must be available and accessible, and, as noted above, they should be inviting. The Surgeon General expressed the belief and the hope that evidence-based practices will reduce the need for coercion in mental health services. He encouraged multiple "portals of entry" to services by creating incentives for many service providers to receive referrals and accept all individuals seeking services (1,14).

Subsequently, individuals can be matched with appropriate evidence-based services that are provided by specially trained clinicians, teams, and programs within the service system. Not every service provider will offer all the evidence-based services, but every clinician and provider organization should offer choices of some of the evidence-based services that are delivered in their organization or elsewhere in the system. There should be no "wrong door" for services. Awareness of evidence-based practices and of where such services can be received is essential information for the contemporary mental health service system.

Reduce financial barriers to treatment

No single policy issue received more attention from the authors of the papers in the evidence-based practices series than the adequacy of financing. Realistically, a service is not available if a person with a mental illness cannot afford to use it or a program cannot afford to provide it for the price offered by payers. It is a simple truism that a service system runs on its financing policies. If evidence-based practices are not covered services, or if the fees paid are below the cost of providing them, they will not be used.

Until very recently, Medicaid policy almost uniformly discouraged assertive community treatment. Federal block grant regulations have complicated the funding of integrated services for individuals who have co-occurring disorders. Payment for multifamily groups is not always covered or reimbursed adequately. The same may be true for various components of self-managed care. Newer medications may not be on the formulary of a pharmacy benefit plan, or copayments may discourage the use of newer agents. Supported employment may not be reimbursed at a rate that compares favorably with the rate that could be obtained through a sheltered workshop.

These are recurrent issues in every discussion of barriers to implementing evidence-based practices. The remedy is self-evident—remove unreasonable financial barriers. However, these policies are often out of the decision-making purview of the mental health authority. Working on these policies with other agencies has become the standard approach for supporting the implementation of evidence-based practices. Resources must support the transition to evidence-based practices in agencies

Infrastructure with continuity of leadership in implementation is important because of the frequent turnover of state mental health program directors.

that have historically been involved in older practices. It is difficult to be motivated to learn a new practice if the old practice generated the agency's revenues. Policy makers and administrators need the tools to shift funding in a logical and incremental manner from old ways of practice to new ways. They also need the resources—both human and financial—to provide technical assistance or quality oversight to ensure that funds are being spent in new ways rather than in old ways that have new names. Funds are needed to offset the opportunity costs associated with learning a new practice.

By and large, the move to evidence-based practices will not be accompanied by a permanent increase in resources. Many successful implementations have occurred when agencies have switched from an older practice, such as brokering case management or rehabilitation-oriented day treatment, to a new practice, such as assertive community treatment or supported employment. These agencies benefit from additional one-time-only resources to support the transition to evidence-based practices.

Implementation might be enhanced by better planning among the agencies responsible for financing care—federal, state, and local authorities—to develop the necessary incentives for implementing and sustaining evidence-based practices. To provide adequate financing, planners also need accurate information about the costs of providing evidence-based services. As with other aspects of the research, cost data from experimental studies often are not generalizable to usual care settings. Cutting across all these courses of action is the need for informed leadership from mental health policy makers and administrators—and increasingly from other sectors, such as Medicaid, the criminal justice system, vocational rehabilitation services, and the education system.

Most authors of the papers in the series indicated the need for a dedicated individual and for infrastructure to support the implementation of evidence-based practices. Infrastructure with continuity of leadership in implementation is important because of the frequent turnover of state mental health program directors. This type of infrastructure is also important in efforts to move from research or pilot projects to systemwide implementation. What may be conceptualized by a clinical or policy leader in an administrative office and supported in the throes of change may become compromised when multiple practitioners or providers or multiple locations are involved.

Infrastructure is needed not only to provide assistance for both leaders and implementers to sustain changing practices but also to change again as new evidence emerges. This capacity for managing change is often not present in public-sector settings that are buffeted by the political or public priority of the day. The necessary research and resources—for training, ongoing support, and travel—to move from a pilot project to full-scale implementation are needed if evidence-based practices are to be implemented broadly and sustained over time with at least a modicum of fidelity.

Infrastructure to support systemic change

Without a template to guide them, various mental health authorities have developed similar infrastructure to support systemic change toward evidence-based practice and quality improvement. Leadership is critical for sorting through all the treatment recommendations and guidelines that are being promoted by various organizations and for developing an evidence standard for assessing practice. Agencies such as the Substance Abuse and Mental Health Services Administration, the National Institute of Mental Health (NIMH), and the Agency for Healthcare Research and Quality as well as foundations such as the Robert Wood Johnson Foundation and the MacArthur Foundation have supported these efforts. Organizations such as the National Association of State Mental Health Program Directors (NASMHPD) and its research institute and the National Alliance for the Mentally Ill (NAMI) have established initiatives and partnerships to promote evidence-based practices.

The Evidence-Based Practices Project began in New Hampshire, Maryland, and Ohio and has spread to several other states. Each of these three states developed its own center for implementing evidence-based practices, taking advantage of local opportunities and preferences. Each state has created its own model and priority practices for implementation. The project has stimulated some cross-fertilization, so the centers share many of the same functions, but the differences are illustrative and might encourage other states to develop similar centers of their own. Each center is sponsored at least in part by the state mental health authority.

Each center views its mission as supporting the implementation of evidence-based practices, which involves training, supervision, ongoing clinical and administrative support in the new practice, and structural support with regulations and financing technical assistance. Each of the centers sponsors needs assessment activities, training events, and various services that support the implementation of evidence-based practices. The centers work with all the stakeholders—the state and local mental health authorities, program administrators, clinicians and other providers, and consumers and their families.

In New Hampshire, the West Institute for Implementing Evidence-Based Practices is a partnership between the state and a private family foundation. The institute grew out of the well-established public-academic linkage between the state mental health authority and Dartmouth Medical School. It is affiliated with the New Hampshire–Dartmouth Psychiatric Research Center, where several of the evidence-based practices were developed and evaluated. The Evidence-Based Practices Project is run out of the West Institute and the New Hampshire–Dartmouth Psychiatric Research Center. The centralized model in New Hampshire is well suited to a small state with a single academic center.

In Maryland, the Center for Implementing Evidence-Based Practices is a newly established center within the Maryland Mental Health Service Improvement Collaborative. Sponsored by the state mental health authority, the center is an outgrowth of the original collaborative that has been devoted to providing training and conference opportunities for service providers in Maryland. Like the New Hampshire center, the Maryland center is a key element of one of the oldest public-academic liaisons in the country, between the department of psychiatry at the University of Maryland and the Mental Hygiene Administration. The specific link is with the Center for Mental Health Services Research, which together with the Johns Hopkins University includes the NIMH-funded research center that conducted the Schizophrenia Patient Outcomes Research Team (PORT) study.

The PORT study was one of the first to identify and explore the major problem of the disparity between research and practice (1,15). No private funds have yet been obtained to support the center, but a network grant from the MacArthur Foundation to the university may fund pilot research on implementing evidence-based practices in these centers.

In contrast with the centralized model used by New Hampshire and Maryland—both comparatively small states—Ohio uses a decentralized approach. The coordinating centers of excellence are a series of centers—currently eight, but ten are planned—decentralized throughout Ohio. Most are linked to a research-oriented institution, either a university or a private-sector entity, that specializes in one area of evidence-based practice. In Ohio, where there are multiple small research centers and where local mental health authorities are largely autonomous and statutorily responsible for mental health services, the decentralized and specialized approach makes the most sense. Some of Ohio's coordinating centers of excellence focus on practices for which there is substantial research evidence; others focus on important areas such as school-based mental health services that cannot wait for an evidence base to accumulate before some guidance is provided to local mental health authorities.

In Texas, statewide implementation of evidence-based practices has occurred through collaboration with academic centers and stakeholder groups, who advocate for resources, as well as through contractual requirements, including financial sanctions, with local mental health authorities. These collaborations have also resulted in major research initiatives related to the implementation of evidence-based practices.

The NASMHPD and the NASMHPD Research Institute, using a grant from NIMH to advance their research on evidence-based practices, are coordinating these research efforts at the level of the state mental health authority. The NASMHPD Research Institute has created a Center on Evidence-Based Practices, Performance Measurement, and Quality

Improvement to support state efforts to implement evidence-based practices and to monitor the quality and impact of the services being provided.

The functions of the center are to identify, share, and promote knowledge about evidence-based practices, performance measurement, and quality improvement; conduct research and develop knowledge; provide technical assistance; and coordinate activities across organizational entities and levels of government. Several other states are involved in the project and have their own approaches to infrastructure development. Private entities, such as the nonprofit Institute of the Technical Assistance Collaborative, are emerging to provide technical assistance related to infrastructure and policies to support evidence-based practices.

Conclusions

The time has come to add to the body of knowledge about implementing evidence-based practices at different levels, including knowledge about policy, program priorities, clinician practice, consumer adherence, and family member support. However, implementation at the policy level is both primary and paramount. The national initiative embodied by the project is one of the most important innovations on the mental health horizon. It will serve as the testing ground for what can be learned about bridging the gap between science and service.

This important initiative will not go far if it is not supported by mental health policies—at state and federal levels—that create the organizational and financial incentives to implement evidence-based practices. In addition, it will be a time-limited activity if it does not also yield lessons about how to adapt to new evidence and ongoing systemic changes. Organizations must be flexible and must be able to learn and adapt.

The promise of decades of research must be realized in practice. The Surgeon General simultaneously identified the promise and documented the shortcomings. His report outlines courses of action for policy makers that should guide us away from service disparities and that support the implementation of evidence-based practices. We have the opportunity to combine quality improvement with accountability through performance measurement and the implementation of effective new services and treatments. ◆

Acknowledgments

Support was provided by grants R24-MH-53148 and P50-MH-43703 from the National Institute of Mental Health and by the Center for Mental Health Services, the Robert Wood Johnson Foundation, and the John D. and Catherine T. MacArthur Foundation.

References

1. Mental Health: A Report of the Surgeon General. Washington, DC, US Department of Health and Human Services, US Public Health Service, 1999

2. Turner JC, TenHoor W: The NIMH community support program: pilot approach to needed social reform. Schizophrenia Bulletin 4:319–348, 1978

3. Morrissey J, Goldman HH: Cycles of reform in the care of the chronically mentally ill. Hospital and Community Psychiatry 35:785–793, 1984

4. Tessler RC, Goldman HH: The Chronically Mentally Ill: Assessing Community Support Programs. Ballinger, Cambridge, Mass, 1982

5. Goldman HH, Morrissey JP, Ridgely MS: Evaluating the program on chronic mental illness. Milbank Quarterly 72:37–48, 1994

6. Bickman L, Guthrie PR, Foster EM: Evaluating Managed Mental Health Care: The Fort Bragg Experiment. New York, Plenum, 1995

7. Torrey W, Drake RE, Dixon L, et al: Implementing evidence-based practices for persons with severe mental illnesses. Psychiatric Services 52:45–50, 2001

8. Briere R: Crossing the Quality Chasm: A New Health System for the 21st Century. Washington, DC, National Academy Press, 2001

9. Rosenberg SD, Mueser KT, Friedman MS, et al: Developing effective treatments for posttraumatic disorders among people with severe mental illness. Psychiatric Services 52:1453–1461, 2001

10. Argyris C: Knowledge for Action: A Guide to Overcoming Barriers to Organizational Change. San Francisco, Jossey-Bass, 1993

11. Lutterman T, Hogan M: State mental health agency controlled expenditures and revenues for mental health services, FY 1981–FY 1998, in Mental Health US, 2000. Rockville, Md, Substance Abuse and Mental Health Services Administration, in press

12. Frese FJ III, Stanley J, Kress K, et al: Integrating evidence-based practices and the recovery model. Psychiatric Services 52:1462–1468, 2001

13. Reiser SJ: Consumer competence and the reform of American health care. JAMA 267:1511–1515, 1992

14. Mental Health: Culture, Race, and Ethnicity: A Supplement to Mental Health: A Report of the Surgeon General. Rockville, Md, US Department of Health and Human Services, 2001

15. Lehman AJ, Steinwachs DM, and the survey co-investigators of the PORT study: Patterns of usual care for schizophrenia: preliminary results from the Schizophrenia Patient Outcomes Research Team (PORT) client survey. Schizophrenia Bulletin 24:11–20, 1998

A Journal for Everyone on the Treatment Team!

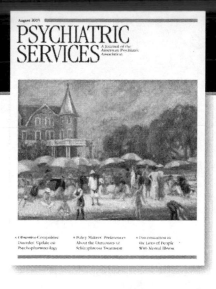 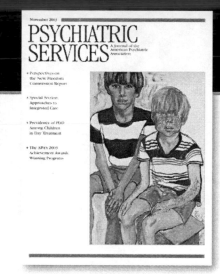 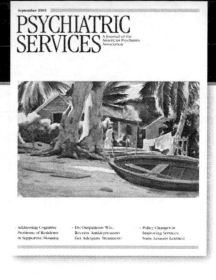

Psychiatric Services is one of the most respected journals in the field of mental health. Each issue is dedicated to disseminating findings on evidence-based practices so that everyone receives the most effective information.

Psychiatric Services addresses every member of the treatment team in its focus on issues related to the delivery of mental health services in organized settings. Each month, it features research reports and commentary on topics at the forefront of psychiatry. Special sections take an in-depth look at a particular psychiatric issue.

With each issue of *Psychiatric Services*, you get:

- Research reports, reviews, and commentary on topics at the forefront of psychiatry
- Columns dealing with topics like the law and psychiatry, geriatrics, economics, psychopharmacology, and alcohol and drug abuse
- Book reviews, news, and letters to the editor
- And much, much more!

A Special Notice for American Psychiatric Association Members

As an APA Member, you are entitled to receive *Psychiatric Services* absolutely FREE. Visit www.appi.org or call 1-800-368-5777 to begin receiving *Psychiatric Services*.

Prices for Non APA Members

Receive both the print and online issues of *Psychiatric Services* for one low price!

US Individuals	$78	International Individuals	$114
US Institutions	$172	International Institutions	$240

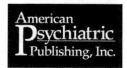

The *First* and *Last* Word in Psychiatry

To order visit our website at **www.appi.org** or call **1-800-368-5777** and refer to priority code **AH401**

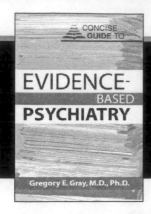

EVIDENCE-BASED PSYCHIATRY

Gregory E. Gray, M.D., Ph.D.

Concise Guide to Evidence-Based Psychiatry is a must-have resource

Concise Guide to Evidence-Based Psychiatry (EBP) is a must-have resource for informed decision-making in psychiatric practice today. This single, easy-to-use reference will enable practitioners to find answers to clinical questions, critically appraise articles, and apply the results of their findings to patients.

This practical handbook provides quick access to EBP theories, tools, and methods. *Concise Guide to Evidence-Based Psychiatry* is a one-stop reference for using the literature to improve patient outcomes.

Features include:

- **Practical**—Filled with how-to information, *Concise Guide to Evidence-Based Psychiatry* outlines the latest techniques for accessing, assessing, and interpreting the literature.

- **Conveniently sized**—Small enough to fit in your jacket pocket, it's ideal for daily reference.

- **Easy to use**—Includes many tables of essential websites for finding reliable information on the Internet, best-practice strategies for searching the medical literature, and critical appraisal worksheets for assessing the validity of findings.

Concise Guide to Evidence-Based Psychiatry fills an important role as the first EBP text for teaching residents, who are now required to develop such skills to meet the ACGME "practice-based learning and improvement" core competency. Special features for pedagogical use include suggestions for teaching EBP in residency programs, profuse examples from the psychiatric literature, and worksheets for the critical appraisal of clinical trials, diagnostic tests, epidemiologic studies, studies of prognosis, and more.

Whether for self-study or use in residency programs, *Concise Guide to Evidence-Based Psychiatry* is the best resource available to help practitioners apply current research findings to their work with patients.

"What a pleasant surprise to find that this very readable book which introduces the principles of evidence-based psychiatry, while offering a brief primer on the basics of statistics, epidemiology and how to critically read the literature. This concise guide manages to be both didactic and practical at the same time, and it transforms a potentially intimidating subject into one within the easy grasp of busy trainees, educators, and clinicians. Its publication is very timely, as the need to teach and learn evidence-based medicine has become an important component of resident education."

—*Ira Lesser, M.D., Director, Residency Training and Vice Chair, Harbor-UCLA Medical Center; Professor, Department of Psychiatry and Biobehavioral Sciences, David Geffen School of Medicine at UCLA*

2004 • 240 pages • ISBN 1-58562-096-3 • paperback • $29.95 • Item #62096

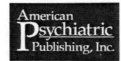

American **Psychiatric** Publishing, Inc.

The *First* and *Last* Word in Psychiatry

To order please visit our website at **www.appi.org** or call **1-800-368-5777** and refer to priority code **AH403**